Ethics and Health Administration: Ethical Decision Making in Health Management

Marc D. Hiller, Dr. P. H.
The University of New Hampshire

Commission on Ethical Issues in Health Management

Association of University Programs in Health Administration

1911 North Fort Myer Drive
Suite 503
Arlington, Virginia 22209

The preparation and publication of this book
was made possible by a grant from the
Pew Memorial Trust

Copyright 1986 by
Association of University Programs in Health Administration,
1911 North Fort Myer Drive, Suite 503
Arlington, Virginia 22209.

Library of Congress Catalog Card No. 86-073245

ISBN 0-910591-00-8

COMMISSION ON ETHICAL ISSUES
IN HEALTH MANAGEMENT

WALTER J. McNERNEY, M.H.A.
(Chairman)
Herman Smith Professor of Hospital and Health
Services Management
J.L. Kellogg Graduate School of Management
Northwestern University
Evanston, Illinois

JOHN C. BEDROSIAN, LL.B.
Senior Executive Vice President
National Medical Enterprise
Los Angeles, California

DANIEL CALLAHAN, Ph.D.
Director, The Hastings Center
Hastings-on-Hudson, New York

EDWARD J. CONNORS
President, Sisters of Mercy Health Corporation
Farmington Hills, Michigan

CHARLES M. EWELL, Ph.D.
President, The Governance Institute
LaJolla, California

ALBERT V. GLOWASKY
Morgan Stanley and Company
New York, New York

MARC D. HILLER, Dr.P.H.
Associate Professor
Department of Health Services Administration and
Policy
University of New Hampshire
Durham, New Hampshire

i

PAMELA MARALDO, R.N., Ph.D.
  Executive Director
  National League for Nursing
  New York, New York

EDMUND D. PELLEGRINO, M.D.
  Director, Kennedy Institute of Ethics
  Georgetown University
  Washington, D.C.

DAVID B. STARKWEATHER, Dr.P.H.
  Professor and Director
  Graduate Program in Health Services Management
  University of California-Berkeley
  Berkeley, California

Project Staff:

David F. Bergwall, D.B.A.
  Vice President, Association of Univerisity Programs
  in Health Administration

Gwen C. Gulesian
  Administrative Assistant, Association of University
  Programs in Health Administration

Contents

PREFACE

Ethical issues have challenged the health field for centuries. In fact, the range and complexity of these issues has helped to make the administration of human services unique. Often situations arise where management principles do not offer help or even apply.

Historically ethical issues in health care have centered around the patient. In today's highly technical, competitive health environment, the number of choices facing care givers and managers has grown dramatically. Often these choices include institutional and community matters and are rooted in the tension between our growing ability to heal and our limited resources to pay the cost of healing.

This monograph comes at an important time. We can no longer send young persons into the field who are unable to deal with ethical questions. We cannot wait for years of hard experience to provide ways of addressing these issues.

The following monograph provides a fundamental grounding in the discipline of ethics and, through excellent examples, applies this discipline to the health institution setting within the content of management. Further, it provides a useful bibliography which assists individuals who wish to reach beyond the scope of this document.

Whereas the Commission designed the monograph with the education of students and faculty in mind, the finished product should provide substantive help to the field of practice. The text can and should be used for in-service training of managers, trustees and other professionals within health services institutions.

Ethics and Health Administration: Ethical Decision Making in Health Management was developed by the Commission on Ethical Issues in Health Management of the Association of University Programs in Health Administration (AUPHA).

v

The activities of the task force were funded over a three-year period by the Pew Memorial Trust, which supported not only this Commission but a related effort on Health Law, as well as general curriculum development for AUPHA. The Trust has been a strong ally in these efforts.

Health administration education is multidisciplinary in structure and content. The building blocks of the professional curriculum reside in a number of disciplines, including management, public health, medicine, political science, law, and their academic subject areas. AUPHA provides leadership to the consortium of its members in melding and shaping the content of these areas into health management curricula.

Assisting universities in curricular development is AUPHA's highest priority. It has conducted a number of highly successful curriculum projects that have significantly altered the scope, content, and quality of health administration education. Previous efforts were primarily responsible for shifting the curriculum from descriptive institutional management to a system wide analytic approach. Other endeavors led to much greater emphasis on the development of quantitative skills, financial management, and planning. The present activity adds still another dimension to curricular development by addressing the ethical issues in the management of health services delivery.

The objectives of the Commission on Ethical Issues in Health Management were:

1. To assess the current state of health administration curricula with regard to managerial ethics;

2. To provide up-to-date guidance on the scope and content of managerial ethics for health administration education and practice;

3. To identify, assemble, and develop needed teaching resources to enhance the breadth and quality of managerial ethics teaching, and;

4. To identify and establish AUPHA's continuing role in relation to managerial ethics in the teaching process.

The Commission examined the current state of health services management curricula with regard to ethics. It discovered an uneven approach across health administration programs and a general lack of systematic coverage of ethics as related to management. Where programs had ethics content it tended to be biomedical rather than management oriented.

Discussions with faculty members lead to the conclusion that few had any formal training in ethics. While many were clearly concerned for the ethical dimension of the curricula, only a few were prepared to address the topic with any rigor. Faculty in health administration programs tend to present antidotal coverage of the topic in a highly individualistic fashion.

The Commission surveyed a selected group of practitioners to identify the ethical issues in management which they face on a daily basis. The little response received indicated a general inability to identify or communicate managerial ethical issues. Again there was a high degree of concern but limited understanding or ability to address problems in an analytic or systematic fashion.

In response to its findings the Commission established the creation of basic teaching materials as its first priority. This monograph was prepared to provide a basic foundation for faculty and practitioners in the discipline of ethics and their application to management decision making in health.

The Commission has identified two major projects for the future.   The first is a casebook which can be used in the classroom as well as in the field of practice. This casebook would focus on issues related to the management of health services delivery organizations and respond to the most frequent request of faculty in the field. The second priority project is the development of faculty fellowships and/or training programs in managerial ethics. The need here is to prepare faculty as "grey area" people to quote Dr. Pellegrino.   These are people who are not ethicists or philosophers but who are trained to address the ethical dimensions of the field.

I would like to thank the Commission members for their strong support, particularly Marc Hiller who graduated from the role of Commissioner to that of principal architect and author.   In behalf of the Commission, I should like to acknowledge the invaluable assistance of AUPHA staff headed by David F. Bergwall.

Walter J. McNerney, M.H.A
(Chairman)
Commission on Ethical Issues
in Health Management

CHAPTER 1

AN INTRODUCTION TO ETHICS IN HEALTH ADMINISTRATION

Try to think of those ten patients as ten ship-
wrecked men on a raft--a raft that is barely
large enough to save them--that will not support
one more. Another head bobs up through the waves
at the side. Another man begs to be taken aboard.
He implores the captain of the raft to save him.
But the captain can only do that by pushing one
of his ten off the raft and drowning him to make
room for the newcomer.

This dramatic scene from George Bernard Shaw's 1911
classic tragedy, *The Doctor's Dilemma*, bears a striking
similarity to the situation facing health care administration today. For even though scientists and physicians
can heal and cure, governing boards and administrators
are increasingly being forced to decide whether cure or
treatment is appropriate, necessary, or even desirable.
There is a bewildering array of options and alternatives
available to the modern health care administrator, many
involving life and death decisions, and the list of medical
and administrative dilemmas seems endless.

During the past few decades, most ethical dilemmas
focused on the physician-patient relationship. Yet many
physicians were ill-prepared to address the problems they
encountered. Medical education was clearly needed to make
doctors more aware of the moral dimensions of their practice. Today, most medical schools have programs to teach
prospective physicians how to address such problems in
a rational, ethical manner.

Ethics think tanks have raised social consciousness
by examining the implications of various medical decisions,
and legislative bodies, professional review boards, and

1

health insurance companies have questioned the burgeoning use of costly new medical procedures before their safety and effectiveness have been evaluated (Stein, 1978, p. 229).

While health administrators have been struggling for years with the ethical problems of institutional management, recent advances in medical technology, limited funds, increasing costs, and competition sharpen the questions posed in *The Doctor's Dilemma*. Following are several examples of the types of decisions facing the modern health care administrator:

> A patient in your hospital needs costly long-term therapy to survive, and the hospital will have to bear the cost. Should you authorize continued treatment if doing so would mean forgoing either needed emergency room renovation or a salary increase for the nursing staff?

> A severely defective newborn is delivered at your hospital. The infant might survive for six months to a year with advanced medical technology. Attending physicians and invited medical consultants support the parents' request to let the baby die without further medical intervention. You, the administrator, are aware of recent federal regulations ("Baby Doe") requiring treatment of handicapped infants. What should you do?

> You are the administrator of the only community hospital within 150 miles. A 38-year-old married businesswoman and her husband, who have three teenage children, come to your office seeking an abortion. The woman says that the doctors on your medical staff have refused her request because of their religious beliefs. No formal institutional policy exists on this issue. What are you going to tell her?

An understanding of ethical theory and principles does not guarantee that one will make the correct decisions, but it does provide an analytical means by which to examine the problem and the value choices.

It is no longer always easy to distinguish between life and death, and expectations about what can be done to forestall death often go beyond rational limits. Such herculean curative powers have created ever more complex ethical dilemmas for health professionals, particularly administrators, since it is they who must juggle competing claims for resources. Unfortunately, many administrators must make choices without being aware that there are rational bases for such decision making.

The health care system is also changing. Government intervention in and regulation of the system and its institutions have decreased markedly in recent years. Public support of health manpower training, medical research, hospital construction and renovation, and health and human services for the aged and poor has also diminished, sometimes to the point of elimination, as has institutional support by private philanthropy. As a result, health care has been increasingly managed by the private sector. The once charitable mission of health care institutions (Rosner, 1982) is being threatened by a trend characterized by the corporatization of health care. The historical humanistic model of health care delivery is being replaced by an economic model that stresses competition and profit.

In a struggle to survive, voluntary community hospitals are behaving more like profit-making businesses and are emphasizing strong business skills. Both investor-owned and nonprofit health care institutions are forming complex multi-institutional arrangements to maximize their financial positions, and, as a result, the traditional care-before-cost philosophy seems to have become history.

As a result of these socioeconomic, political, and technological influences, administrators are expected to design innovative strategic plans, ward off competition, increase market share, capture new sources of capital while maintaining the old, and, above all, improve the "bottom line." In addition, institutions are expected to ensure

3

equitable access to care. In short, administrators have reached an ethical imperative in the midst of what Starr (1982) has described as nothing less than a "social transformation of American medicine."

* * *

This monograph comprises three papers that students and practitioners of health administration, who are now or will eventually be responsible for solving ethical dilemmas, should find helpful. The first paper provides an overview of ethics and values. It is intended as a primer for those who have not engaged in a formal study of ethics or its application in decision making. The second paper focuses on ethical decision making and health administration and is more practical than theoretical. It is designed to help administrators identify different types of ethical problems and conflicts, distinguish these from legal questions, and actually engage in the process of ethical analysis. The third paper identifies a wide range of specific ethical issues confronting health administrators and explores various approaches to their study. It also examines the many sources of ethical conflict and provides a broad grouping of ethical issues arising in health administration.

Certain fundamental positions are assumed. First, ethical issues confronting an institution cannot be resolved in isolation from the people who work there. The physicians, nurses, managers, board members, and other staff, all of whom hold an obligation to the institution and its clients, are deeply involved in these issues and their resolution. However, discussions of ethics that affect the institution itself must transcend the values and beliefs of individuals and reflect the institution as its own moral agent.

Second, those charged with overseeing the moral mission of an institution bear a unique role. They must ensure the institution's economic viability in order to keep its doors open, and at the same time they must serve a social good. Administrators must thus learn to recognize and address the many ethical dilemmas that result from this dual mission (Hiller and Gorsky, 1986).

Third, reliance on "gut" reactions and other informal approaches to solving ethical dilemmas are inadequate. Health administrators frequently find themselves balanced on a high wire surrounded by competing demands and expectations, with no net below them. All around are conflicting accountabilities: social/community, corporate/owner, consumer/patient, resource, regulatory, and third party (Austin, 1974, p. 16). Indeed, the range and degree of moral dilemmas confronting health care management have never been greater.

References

Austin, Charles J. "What is health administration?" *Hospital Administration* 19:14-29, Summer 1974.

Hiller, Marc D., and Robin D. Gorsky. "Shifting priorities and values: a challenge to the hospital's mission." In George J. Agich and Charles E. Begley, eds., *The Price Of Health: Economics and Ethics in Medicine.* Boston, Mass.: D. Reidel Publishing Company, 1986.

Rosner, David. *A Once Charitable Enterprise: Hospitals and Health Care in Brooklyn and New York, 1885-1915.* New York: Cambridge University Press, 1982.

Starr, Paul. *The Social Transformation of American Medicine.* New York: Free Press, 1982.

Stein, Jane J. *Making Medical Choices: Who Is Responsible?* Boston, Mass.: Houghton Mifflin Company, 1978.

CHAPTER 2

THE DISCIPLINE OF ETHICS

ETHICS, MORALS, AND VALUES

Ethics is the branch of philosophy dealing with systematic approaches to understanding morality. Its roots are in ancient Greece and the teachings of Plato and Aristotle. It is the disciplined study of the nature and justification of moral principles, decisions, and problems.

Ethics determines norms, standards of behavior (or practice), or guidelines that apply to the judgment of human acts. Ethics does not dictate specific answers; it is neither empirical nor absolute. Philosophers and theologians who study ethics, commonly referred to as ethicists, try to understand morality systematically. They analyze conflict and attempt to understand why certain types of acts or behavioral characteristics are considered morally "better" than others (Purtilo and Cassel, 1981, p. 5). According to Beauchamp and McCullough (1984, p. 11), they

> seek a reasoned defense for a system of norms
> of conduct from a comprehensive and coherent
> moral point of view. Through the medium of moral
> principles, philosophers try to distinguish a
> good moral claim--one that can be justified in
> terms of principles, from a bad moral claim--one
> that cannot be justified in terms of principles.
> To this end, philosophers try to exhibit how
> not to confuse a merely personal attitude or
> intuition--i.e., unreflective and nonobjective
> "principles"--with a reasoned and justified moral
> position.

Beauchamp and McCullough continue by arguing that "One must have defensible moral reasons for holding a position, and neither the position nor the reasons that underlie it can be justified if they rest solely on prejudice, emotion, false data, the authority of another individual, or claims of self-evidence." This is a crucial point because ethical principles provide reasons for action that transcend individual beliefs. Since ethical principles can pull in multiple, or conflicting, directions, however, they cannot always be expected to lead to simple resolution of moral problems. Rather, they inherently promote further in-depth questioning and rejustification of options and help to ensure adherence to a well-planned approach that considers both the basis for decisions and the process by which decisions are made.

More simply, ethics attempts to find good reasons for holding certain values or adopting certain principles or duties as a guide to decision making. It also attempts to provide a rational foundation for arbitrating disputes; balancing conflicting ethical principles, values, and obligations; and establishing priorities.

In contrast, *morals* reflect traditions of belief about right and wrong often associated with a particular religion or social consensus. Morality is a social institution with a history and code of learnable rules, and people are taught as they mature to mold to these rules and traditions. Morality is a product of social consensus over a long period of time, and it often differs from actions grounded in or precipitated by emotion, prejudice, or personal interest (Beauchamp and Bowie, 1983, p. 1).

Pellegrino and Thomasma (1981, p. 179) contend that the word *moral* refers to any action involving values and that no judgment or comparison of values is implied. Thus, reference to medicine or health care management as a moral enterprise merely means that decisions made by those in these professions are value-laden. Thus, the conscious and unconscious influence of personal and professional values in the decision-making process cannot be denied.

Values constitute the worth or merit that an individual or society places on something, regardless of standards, principles, or norms. Values reflect a wide range of personal beliefs, experiences, culture, and religion. Many

8

decisions are based on value-laden factors rather than on clear moral standards or ethical principles. In view of the extent to which values may influence health care decisions, particularly in our complex health care system and pluralistic society, the importance of values clarification should never be minimized or denied.

Some people are unaware of their own values and the influence of these values on what they do. It is easy to recognize positive values that go along with high moral standards, but others--both positive and negative--may not be as obvious, although they still influence decision making, albeit unconsciously. Values clarification is a process by which people sort through, analyze, and assign priorities to their values. It provides the individual an opportunity to separate personal and professional values and permits a better understanding of why and how one is led toward making certain types of decisions--for better or worse--thereby allowing rational intervention. While values clarification can help in personal growth, it is strictly nonnormative and nonprescriptive. It is likely that an individual will act in accord with his or her values; nonetheless, decisions should be made in accord with fundamental normative ethical principles.

DESCRIPTIVE ETHICS, METAETHICS, AND NORMATIVE ETHICS

Three approaches dominate the literature of ethics and ethical theory. Two, descriptive ethics and metaethics, attempt to describe and analyze morality without assuming a position. The third, normative ethics, assumes moral positions and appeals to a body of ethical theory in doing so. Although these categories are not mutually exclusive and frequently overlap, it is helpful to understand certain distinctions.

Descriptive ethics is the factual investigation and explanation of moral behavior and beliefs. Sociologists, anthropologists, psychologists, and historians assess moral codes, attitudes, and beliefs. For example, a study describing how health administrators as a group view treatment of the terminally ill falls into this category.

Metaethics, a conceptual view of ethics, is concerned with determining the underlying reasons for making moral judgments. It involves the analysis of the meanings of important ethical terms such as "right," "obligation," "virtue," and "responsibility." It asks the underlying question "Why is an act considered moral or immoral?" Whereas descriptive ethics attempts to define that which is factual, metaethics attempts to describe that which is conceptually true. Neither provides prescriptive guides for decision making or action.

In contrast, *normative ethics* asks concrete questions and attempts to determine which acts are morally acceptable. For example, it attempts to assess "the morally praise-worthy/blameworthy traits of persons or institutions" (Purtilo and Cassel, 1981, p. 5). In other words, normative ethics seeks to determine what *ought to be* done rather than what *is* done and is therefore prescriptive (Beauchamp and Bowie, 1983, p. 6; Beauchamp and Childress, 1983, p. 8). Rooted in ethical theory, normative ethics formulates and defends systems of fundamental ethical principles and rules that determine whether an action is right or wrong. Ideally, an ethical theory would be complete and universally valid, but many questions remain unanswered simply because of life's complexities (Beauchamp and Childress, 1983, p. 8).

APPLYING ETHICS

Applied ethics constitutes the application of normative ethical principles and reasoning to either specific ethical issues such as abortion, corporate responsibility, or euthanasia, or problems that arise in particular professions such as medicine, engineering, journalism, jurisprudence, business, or health administration. In general, the same ethical principles apply to most professional problems.

Applied ethics has become popular in the past decade, judging from the number of courses in many professional schools. In a recent study conducted by the Hastings Center, Callahan (1980, p. 2) reported,

> Almost every medical school in the country has initiated at least some introduction to medical ethics. . . . Almost 90 percent of law schools require courses in professional responsibility. Courses on corporate responsibility are emerging in business and accounting schools. Major programs in applied ethics are appearing in schools of nursing, of journalism, and of engineering; and there are other specialized courses in environmental ethics and the ethics of social science research, public policymaking, and administration.

Whether as a result of major technological innovations, such as in medicine, or the dramatic change in the social context in which professionals operate, the number of moral dilemmas is increasing. "Conflicts of interest, whistle blowing on corruption, obligations to clients or patients versus duties to society, and the consequences of deception versus truth-telling" (Callahan, 1980, p. 2) are common sources of ethical problems.

Callahan (1980, p. 1) notes that applied ethics provides "a strategy for fostering professional responsibility" by developing reasoning capacity in five ways:

1. Stimulation of moral imagination. Applied ethics teaches that all decisions bear certain consequences and that all moral choices have a variety of implications. Since all human actions may reflect a moral point of view, no decision can be dismissed as "strictly professional."

2. Recognition of ethical issues. Applying ethics encourages individuals to examine their responses to and assumptions about decisions influenced by value elements. It forces them to compare their immediate responses to responses made after ethical deliberation and can also

11

help in distinguishing ethical questions from political and economic ones.

3. Development of analytical skills. Applied ethics requires an understanding of fundamental ethical principles and rules so they can be consistently and coherently applied to problems. It also helps develop sound arguments.

4. Promotion of a sense of moral responsibility. Ethics generates a sense of moral responsibility, strengthening the connection between ethical behavior and personal conduct. Moreover, it fosters individual freedom to make moral choices.

5. Tolerance and resolution of disagreement. Applying ethics does not guarantee that problems will be solved. Rather, it increases tolerance of differences and minimizes the tendency to label others' choices as unethical or immoral. Through identification and clarification of such differences, however, applied ethics helps resolve disagreements through further analysis.

Level of Application

A major difficulty in applying ethics in health administration is distinguishing among individual administrators, the profession of health administration (composed of individual health administrators), and the institutions to which administrators are accountable. While each manager inevitably holds a set of personal and professional values and thereby attempts to administer an institution in an ethical manner, some argue that an institution itself must serve as a moral agent, which implies that ethics can be applied to institutions as well as to individuals.

While not much has been written about institutional ethics (versus professional ethics, to which individual administrators are expected to adhere), Pellegrino and Thomasma (1981) maintain that hospitals, as well as other health care organizations, bear collective moral obliga-

12

tions. They further claim that a hospital's paramount
obligation is to the patient:

> A hospital, by the very fact of its existence
> in a community, makes a declaration; that is,
> it professes to concentrate and make available
> those resources which a person can call upon
> if he is ill. Implicit in that profession is
> the promise to assist the sick person to regain
> what he has lost--his health--at least to the
> maximum degree possible. Thus the profession
> of the hospital is analogous to the profession
> of individual health care providers. (pp. 250-251)

> It seems clear that institutionalization of so
> many aspects of medicine places the hospital
> increasingly in a moral relationship with the
> patient not too different from the doctor's.
> This means a great deal more than simply providing
> the setting in which medicine can be practiced
> safely and competently as well as assuring its
> managerial efficiency and fiscal integrity, though
> these too are obligations. What is called for
> is a sharing of the same range of ethical respon-
> sibilities which have traditionally been implicit
> in the relationship between the physician and
> patient. The board of trustees must feel moral
> as well as legal responsibility for the actions
> of the professional and nonprofessional workers
> within its walls. This responsibility, even
> in presumably professional matters, cannot be
> delegated. Institutional morality, by necessity,
> must concern itself with every facet of the cor-
> porate life of that institution. The result
> is an overlap and sharing of moral obligations
> in which the professional and the institution
> check and balance each other more intimately
> than is now customary. (pp. 252-253)

Thus, Pellegrino and Thomasma argue that institutions hold
ethical responsibilities and are obligated to uphold funda-

mental ethical principles in a manner similar to administrators.

Health care institutions may be moral agents bound by a set of common fundamental ethical principles, but they are not human beings. The collective moral responsibility of the institution must be assumed by those within it (DeGeorge, 1982, p. 90). Whether responsibility is centered on a single chief executive officer or an executive committee, or distributed throughout the organization in a decentralized management model, it rests with administration. Thus, administrators are obligated to adhere to their own personal and professional values as well as to exercise the collective moral responsibility of the institution. When the values at hand are shared, the task is difficult; when values conflict, it becomes an overwhelming challenge demanding considerable skill in ethical analysis.

Apart from the institution, one must also focus on health administration as a profession. Austin (1974, p. 1) suggests that "Health administration is unique, both as a specialty field of administration and as a function within the health and medical care industry; health administration may be viewed theoretically in a systems context but must also be looked at as an emerging profession that is taking on the attributes as well as the self-limiting features of professionalism."

Health administration seems a somewhat hybrid profession, however. While rooted in the charitable healing mission of medicine, it also embraces many business concepts, management principles, and practices. Because of this duality, it is difficult to apply ethics to its unique problems. For example, administrators with a business background often mean something different from those with a health care background when using the word *ethics*. In the business sector, ethics often appears to be interpreted "as a code word for a set of rules of correct conduct, in the sense of things one must do in order to avoid trouble with the law or with one's associates" (Beauchamp and Bowie, 1983, p. 6). Some business people believe that ethics

14

should not be a public matter; it should remain in-house. However, administrators with a strong grounding in health care often appear to have a greater sense of social and ethical obligations that extends beyond purely legal obligations. Such differences create difficulties, but the schisms appear to be thinning as the profession matures.

ETHICAL THEORIES AND PRINCIPLES

A well-developed ethical theory provides a framework for application of and adherence to fundamental principles that guide decision making and action. In recent years, three types of theories have received most of the attention: utilitarian, deontological, and virtue theories.

Utilitarian theories attempt to measure the worth of actions by their ends and consequences and are thus sometimes called consequentialist or teleologic theories. Their classical origins are found in the works of David Hume, Jeremy Bentham, and John Stuart Mill. Mill's *Utilitarianism* (1974) is generally accepted as the treatise on the subject. In it, Mill proposes that the principle of utility should be the foundation of normative ethical theory. Utilitarianism "Is rooted in the thesis that an action or practice is right (when compared to any alternative action or practice) if it leads to the greatest possible balance of good consequences or to the least possible balance of bad consequences" (Beauchamp and Bowie, 1983, p. 21). It holds that individual goods, or rights, are to be surrendered for the common, or collective, good. In so doing, it promotes human welfare by maximizing benefits and minimizing harms. Somewhat ironically, the most common criticism of utilitarianism is that in attempting to provide "the greater good for the greatest number," it can lead to harm or injustice for a minority.

In contrast, deontological, or formalist, theories hold that while good consequences are important, other factors must also be considered. Supporters contend that an ethical theory must be duty-based rather than consequential. The large number of deontological theories often

15

compete with each other as well as with utilitarian theories.

The roots of deontology are diverse and include some religious ethics that concentrate on divine commands. The key point, however, is that at least some acts are wrong or right, independent of their consequences.

Immanuel Kant's ethical theory is often viewed as the first unambiguous formulation of deontology. He said that actions should be based on duty--nothing else--and insisted that all persons act not only "in accordance with duty" but "for the sake of duty." In other words, one's motive must always be grounded in duty or obligation. Kant further argues that it is not enough for one to merely perform morally correct acts if they are based solely on acting in one's self-interest. Self-interest has nothing to do with morality or ethical behavior (Beauchamp and Bowie, 1983, p. 34).

Kant's categorical imperative states that persons must be treated as ends in themselves and never solely as means to the ends of others. Moreover, every individual has an "autonomous" will to govern himself in accordance with universally valid moral principles. The importance of motives underlying actions is clear, and exempting oneself from certain things without granting similar privileges to others or acting on the basis of self-interest are clearly immoral (Beauchamp and Bowie, 1983, pp. 34-35).

In his classic analysis, Ross (1930) developed another important deontological theory based on "prima facie duties." In arguing that there are several different sources and types of moral duties not necessarily derived from the principle of utility, he contends that one must find "the greatest duty" in any circumstance by finding "the greatest balance" of right over wrong in that situation.

Ross described a "prima facie duty" as one that must always be acted on unless it conflicts, in a particular situation, with an equal or stronger duty. In other words, a prima facie duty is considered right and binding if all other things are equal. It cannot be overridden or outweighed by competing moral demands. Therefore, one's actual duty is determined by examining the respective weights of competing prima facie duties. Such duties are therefore not absolute (Beauchamp and Bowie, 1983, p. 39). Most prima facie duties can best be expressed in terms of fundamental ethical principles, such as beneficence, nonmaleficence, respect for persons (autonomy), justice, and utility (Beauchamp and McCullough, 1984, pp. 13-14).

Purtilo and Cassel (1981, p. 9) illustrate the distinction between utilitarianism and deontology:

In present U.S. society, there is much concern about the costs of providing ongoing medical care for the terminally ill and the severely disabled. If one looks only at the overall economic consequences for society of providing life-sustaining care, it might make sense to conclude: "Let these people go--they cost too much to maintain." The formalists call attention to a deep-seated moral conviction, held by many members of society, which says that we ought not to allow harm (in this instance, in the forms of death or increased debility) to befall vulnerable members of society just because it costs so much to maintain them at a reasonably humane level of existence. Even at considerable cost the moral 'pull' is to avoid inflicting harm; therefore, solely a consequences-based approach would appear to oversimplify the moral life.

While the example shows how the two theories may appear mutually exclusive, such is not necessarily the case. Although one might tend to value the preservation of life at all costs on the grounds of inflicting no harm, the argument loses credibility if the question of cost is ignored. Because no one can argue persuasively that every life ought to be saved at any cost, the consequence of economic cost must be considered at some point.

Most formalists today agree to some extent with their utilitarian colleagues that consequences ought to be considered, but they maintain that other principles ought not to be overly compromised by focusing only on consequences. For this reason, several hybrid ethical theories (e.g., rule-utilitarianism, act-utilitarianism) that mix features of consequentialism and formalism have evolved, but they are beyond the scope of this discussion.

A third significant group of ethical theories is based on virtues, that is, the goodness or badness of people's moral character. These theories give importance to various character traits, attitudes, and motives such as honesty, compassion, and reasonableness that are more or less universally cherished. Whereas both consequentialist and formalist theories stress judgments based on specific acts committed by individuals, virtue theories emphasize the moral character (i.e., the goodness or the badness) of individuals. In other words, the moral worth of persons, as well as the rightness or wrongness of their acts, is considered (Beauchamp and Childress, 1983, p. 260). While the degree of goodness or badness associated with judgments may vary from person to person and from one society to the next, virtues are embedded in value systems and influence the decisions one makes.

An individual whose decisions are influenced or reflected by virtues is deemed "virtuous." Purtilo and Cassel (1981, p. 6) claim that, in turn, "failure to exhibit these traits and failure to act from such motives or attitudes could cause an individual to be judged (morally) blameworthy or 'unvirtuous.'"

Virtues are acquired habits or dispositions that guide individuals to do what is morally right or praiseworthy without constantly struggling over the rightness or wrongness of each action. In ethical theory, virtues are usually, if not always, correlated with ethical principles. In other words, for every ethical principle, there is one or more corresponding moral virtue or disposition that "makes" persons act in accord with the duties derived from the principle (Beauchamp and McCullough, 1984, p. 17).

18

Hence, an individual may adhere to morally desirable or praiseworthy virtues as a matter of established behavior without constantly struggling to enforce the demands of specific ethical principles.

While we would like to consider everyone virtuous, often physicians and other health professionals have been imbued with more virtue than other members of society. Given the dependence on them, perhaps it is legitimate to believe in their greater-than-ordinary capacity to do good and avoid evil.

According to the theory of virtue, a decision is based on a particular situation and is not necessarily part of a larger principle. Its weakness, therefore, lies in the potential to be inconsistent when a number of decisions are viewed collectively, since each was based on the individual circumstances of a specific case. In other words, there is no precedent for treating all cases the same.

A great deal has been written about a set of fundamental principles that can be applied to ethical problems. Using a simplified hierarchical diagram, Beauchamp and Childress (1983, p. 5) illustrate that moral reasoning involves varying degrees of abstraction and systematization (Table 1). Their discussion helps clarify the application of ethical theories and principles to health care management problems.

Beauchamp and Childress's hierarchy of ethical reasoning includes, from the bottom: specific judgments or actions, rules, principles, and theories. Thus, an action represents a decision. A rule states that an action should or should not be taken because it is right or wrong. For example, "It is wrong to lie to a patient." Principles are more general and fundamental than rules and should form the foundation of most of the rules that govern administrative actions. Theories are bodies of principles and rules used to resolve conflicts between principles. In sum, "judgments about what ought to be done in particular situations are justified by moral rules, which in turn

TABLE 1   Hierarchy of Ethical Reasoning

Theories   Systematically related bodies of princi-
                ples and rules; used to resolve conflicts
                between principles

Principles   Serve as a foundation or source for justi-
                fying rules which guide decision making

Rules   State that actions of a certain kind ought
                (or ought not) to be made because they are
                "right" or "wrong"

Judgments   Constitute specific decisions, verdicts,
(or Actions)   or conclusions

Source: Adopted from Beauchamp and Childress, (1983, p.
5).

are justified by principles, which ultimately are justified
by ethical theories" (Beauchamp and Childress, 1983, p.
5).

While no principle alone can ensure ethical decision
making, together a set of principles can orchestrate a
well-balanced approach to resolving thorny moral dilemmas.
Table 2 summarizes the five fundamental ethical principles
--beneficence, nonmaleficence, respect for persons, justice,
and utility--and highlights their applicability to health
administration.

Beneficence

Beneficence means literally "to benefit." More broad-
ly, "its meanings include the doing of good, the active
promotion of good, kindness, and charity" (Beauchamp and
McCullough, 1984, p. 27). However, when several hundred
people need to be "done good" at the same time, the prag-

matic and often troublesome administrative question becomes: Whose interests hold top priority?

The earliest expression of beneficence in health care is found in the Hippocratic Oath, wherein the central mission of medicine is proclaimed: "I will apply dietetic measures to the benefit of the sick according to my ability and judgment; I will keep them from harm and injustice" (Edelstein, 1943, p. 3). Modern medicine continues to believe that the obligation to benefit patients is primary

TABLE 2   Fundamental Ethical Principles Relevant to Health Administration

Beneficence	The obligation to benefit one's institution and those it serves (e.g., community, patients, staff)
Nonmaleficence	The obligation to bring no harm or injury to one's institution or to those it serves
Respect for Persons (Autonomy)	The obligation to protect and preserve individual autonomy (self-determination) of those affected by administrative decisions and managerial practices, particularly that of patients and staff
Justice	The obligation to act in a fair and impartial manner in making administrative decisions that affect one's institution or any party it serves (e.g., in allocating or rationing limited resources and/or services, benefits or burdens, risks and costs)
Utility	The obligation to balance the above principles to maximize the greatest utility in administrative decision making

(Amundsen, 1978). But there are wider ramifications. For example, if a physician acts only for the patients' benefit, others might be harmed, including the institution.

Beneficence has a broader and more difficult set of obligations for health administrators. In accord with the hospital's historical healing mission, administrators are obligated to benefit not only the patients in their institution but also the institution itself and the community it serves. Providing the best possible treatment to all in need of care has been the hospital's foremost responsibility since the founding of the Pennsylvania Hospital in 1751 (McGibony, 1969, p. 95).

More recently, events have forced administrators to address the increasing need to ensure institutional survival. In doing so, it becomes paramount that they remain sensitive to the healing mission. At times, administrators indirectly benefit patients by doing that which is best for the institution so that the institution is able to increase its service to patients and the community. In cases where dual institutional missions exist, administrators must wrestle with conflicts (e.g., the patient versus the institution) that arise as a result of overwhelming available resources. In such cases, administrators must choose one over the other—often a clear ethical dilemma (Ginzberg, 1984).

There are other responsibilities as well, not the least of which is increasing institutional efficiency and revenue production. Such drives are often magnified by (but not limited to) the growing for-profit sector of the industry. Some believe that the proprietary sector values profit over healing and caring, thereby skewing the "beneficent" advantage toward stockholders rather than patients (Cunningham, 1982, 1983).

Scholars such as Pellegrino (1978, 1981, 1985), O'Rourke (1984), Young (1984, 1985), Relman (1980, 1985), and Starr (1982) have argued that the healing mission must reign supreme; if it is sacrificed to economic or entrepreneurial interests, beneficence and justice will be com-

22

promised. Others, such as Wikler (1985), have offered a more moderate opinion; and those who support health care for profit have disagreed (Sloan and Vraciu, 1983; Rosett, 1984; Williams, 1984).

The principle of beneficence maintains that administrators ought to make decisions that best support the mission of their institution regardless of ownership. Moreover, it calls for kindness and goodness in administrative actions involving employees. Administrative policies, decisions, and practices should reflect institutional beneficence and benefit staff as long as the primary institutional mission is not compromised.

Nonmaleficence

Nonmaleficence prohibits doing harm. It requires that health administrators avoid misconduct and wrongdoing that could result in harm or injury to associates, staff, and patients. It also establishes a minimum level of beneficence; that is, if one is unable to do good, then one must at least do no harm.

An administrator is obligated to avoid harming his or her institution no matter how unlikely that might be, and to ensure that no harm is knowingly caused to patients or employees. While nonmaleficence most often establishes what ought not to be done, it incurs an obligation to ensure that staff is competent and that all necessary safety and security precautions have been taken.

Nonmaleficence spawns many rules of administrative behavior, such as those obligating sound quality assurance programs, reasonable personnel policies (e.g., salaries, continuing education, and grievance procedures), and business practices that minimize harm.

23

Respect for Persons (Autonomy)

Autonomy dictates that all persons deserve respect and dignity, reflecting Kant's belief that no one should ever be treated only as a means to another's ends. Administrators are thus obligated to ensure a certain level of respect and dignity when ordering others to perform odious tasks or even to serve primarily as the means to another's end. For example, it is permissible to ask someone to scrub floors or empty bedpans if one provides satisfactory working conditions and a decent salary. Such workers deserve respect as persons regardless of the tasks they are asked to perform.

Administrators are bound by this principle to ensure independence and self-governance to patients and staff as long as they neither threaten nor harm another. Engaging in actions that limit independence or deny the right to self-determination is prohibited by autonomy.

Autonomy also provides guidance and direction for more specific rules that address situations in which respect for persons could be compromised. "To every degree possible the autonomy of persons, primarily patients, should be preserved and protected. It is applicable in numerous administrative decisions growing out of patient care activities by doctors and nurses" (Starkweather, 1986, p. 4).

Autonomy should provide a foundation for institutional policies and guidelines governing a wide array of sensitive issues affecting both staff and patients, such as decisions to forgo life-sustaining care, treatment or non-treatment of defective newborns, organ acquisition and transplantation, human experimentation, confidentiality and privacy, and informed consent. While many view such issues as solely within the purview of the physician-patient relationship, administrators must assume responsibility for establishing and adhering to institutional policies and guidelines to protect patients.

Sound management requires that administrators respect everyone with whom they deal: board members, professional and nonprofessional staff, government agencies, stockholders, and the community at large. Doing so requires at all times telling the truth, avoiding deception, ensuring informed consent for all patient services (including the disclosures of the potential charge for those services), and being honest in advertising and marketing. The administrator must also ensure that differences of opinion or outright conflict between caregivers and managers, who must impose staffing limitations, do not create a loss of respect for those who disagree with management. This also holds true for interaction with patients. While disagreements over charges, billing procedures, and other financial matters are inevitable, administrators have an obligation to discuss them openly and honestly.

Strong advocates of autonomy are quick to use it to defend personal liberty, which sometimes must be tempered and restrained in situations where harm might come to others. More debatable, as in some recent cases involving patient refusal of treatment or suicide attempts, is what action to take when only the person seeking liberty of action is harmed. Situations involving incompetents are also a source of conflict.

Justice

Justice is probably the most complex fundamental ethical principle, and possibly the most important in administrative decision making. Indeed, many of the thorniest ethical problems in health care management involve principles of justice. This entails fairness and impartiality and has been closely linked with the concept of just deserts.

The concepts of distributive justice and material justice are most germane to health administration. Distributive justice refers to the justified distribution or allocation of societal benefits and burdens. A burden is both the direct and indirect costs associated with health care, such as the direct payment for hospital care or taxation to support Medicare or Medicaid.

25

While most societies state that all persons are of equal worth and often support this claim through various legal guarantees, economic and political differences or inequities among individuals abound. Discussions revolving around issues of distributive justice therefore typically reflect how to fairly distribute specific limited resources such as health care (Telfer, 1976).

In addressing concepts of material justice, a rather minimal principle most often associated with Aristotle provides the foundation: equals ought to be treated equally and unequals may be treated unequally. The problem with this formal, or "root," principle is its lack of substance or direction. It fails to prescribe how equality should be determined and offers no specific criteria for it. For example, who is equal and who is unequal? On what basis should individuals be compared? For this reason, material justice cannot guide conduct.

Philosophers have competed to develop and defend a wide array of rival material justice principles, sometimes referred to as theories of justice, all of which are compatible with the root principle. Each attempts to illustrate a means by which justice can apply to or be assured in specific situations. In other words, "each material principle of justice identifies a relevant property on the basis of which burdens and benefits should be distributed. Each principle is made a plausible candidate by the relevance of the property it isolates" (Beauchamp and Childress, 1983, p. 187).

Beauchamp and Bowie (1983, p. 42) list six principles of material justice:

1. to each person an equal share,
2. to each person according to individual need,
3. to each person according to that person's rights,
4. to each person according to individual effort,

5. to each person according to societal
    contribution,
6. to each person according to merit.

Any one of these material principles will systematically
explain a particular theory of justice, and the authors
acknowledge that some theories accept all six as valid.

Most societies have adopted several theories because
they believe that different rules apply to different situations, and depending on the moral argument, the priority
of one over another may change. Egalitarian theories of
justice emphasize equal access to primary goods; Marxist
theories emphasize need; libertarian theories are based
on rights to social and economic liberty (implicitly in-
voking criteria of merit and contribution to society);
and utilitarian theories use mixed criteria to obtain the
greatest possible public and private good.

The principle of equal share (egalitarianism) is fairly
straightforward. It advocates that available resources,
regardless of their scarcity, ought to be divided equally.
Two of the most common types of egalitarian theories are
those advocating a right to equal access to health care
supported by Outka (1974), Veatch (1976, 1979), and Childress (1979) and those endorsing entitlement to a decent
minimum supported by Fried (1976) and by Beauchamp and
Faden (1979).

Since equal access to health care does not mean that
everyone will get the same care regardless of need, its
supporters use qualifiers to defend it. The decent minimum
approach also causes difficulties because no one can agree
on what ought to constitute a "decent minimum," particularly
in an era of such rapid technological progress.

The principle of need states that just (i.e., fair
or deserved) distribution is based on fundamental or essential need, without which a person will be harmed. However,
it is difficult to define need and usually depends on who
is doing the defining. As a result, need is often inter-

preted using only medical criteria determined by physicians.

The theory of justice based on societal contribution argues that some members of society deserve more than others because they have contributed (or most likely will contribute) more to society or other persons (e.g., family members). Thus, decision makers are put in the position of having to judge individuals' worthiness (Hiller, 1984, p. 154).

A libertarian theory of justice emphasizes the right of individuals to enter and withdraw freely from arrangements as they choose. It argues that because people freely choose the economic arrangements to which they contribute, it is morally justifiable to distribute scarce health care resources (as well as other economic burdens and benefits) to some and not to others.

Libertarians believe that only minimal government is necessary to protect fundamental rights. However, since some groups have more power in the marketplace than others, libertarianism appears to favor some groups over others. The chief proponent of the theory is Robert Nozick (1974). Sade (1971) also defends a strict libertarian view on the grounds that a right to health care violates physicians' rights to determine when, how, and for what price patients will be treated.

While most people acknowledge that some government intervention (e.g., Medicaid, Medicare) is necessary to ensure equal access to health care, allocation of that care has been influenced significantly by other principles of justice. Beauchamp and Childress (1983, p. 190) state that "The United States has largely, though not exclusively, operated on the principle that distributions of health care services and goods are best left to the marketplace, where the implicit distributive principle is ability to pay. This marketplace principle relies upon some form of libertarian theory of justice for its justification." Now that the American health care industry is increasingly being privatized and operated for profit, libertarians, and their ability-to-pay theory of justice, are becoming more prominent.

If one is to join the debate about the moral implications of health care for profit, one must adopt one principle of justice over another. Such a trend may mean increasing evidence of explicit or implicit diminution of access for the poor, which can be argued as fundamentally unjust. Those who support for-profit health care have publicly denied that such a move decreases access to care and therefore refuse to see it as unjust. Others believe the opposite, and some data support this, but no conclusions have been drawn.

Denial of something to which one is entitled is unjust, but the debate still rages over whether health care is a right (of individuals), or conversely, an obligation (of, for example, government, health care institutions, or physicians). While opinions differ, most legal scholars agree that there is a limited and definable legal right to health care in the United States. However, no one can agree about how to establish a hierarchy or level of such rights.

From the broader philosophical perspective, arguments favoring social justice and individual rights more clearly explicate the presence of an undeniable moral right, or claim, to health care according to various material principles of justice. In turn, economics has contributed significantly toward the development of theories of distributive justice. Thus, two important economic terms need definition: *microallocation*, which describes decisions about which individuals ought to receive available resources, and *macroallocation*, which describes decisions about which resources society ought to make available.

Kass (1971, p. 779) illustrates the wide spectrum of decisions. Personnel and facilities for medical research and treatment are scarce resources. Is development of new technology the best use of those resources, and how should efforts aimed at prevention be balanced against those aimed at cure, or either effort against attempts

29

to redesign the species? How should delivery of available care be balanced against further basic research? And what should be done about eliminating poverty, pollution, urban decay, discrimination, and poor education?   This last question is perhaps the most profound.

In general, physicians and other clinicians are involved mostly in microallocation issues, such as which of two patients should be placed on the single available respirator or given the only available donor organ. Public policymakers, on the other hand, more often focus on macroallocation issues, such as to what extent medical care ought to be guaranteed by the government or how resources should be divided among medical research, medical education, hospital construction, and direct care. They are concerned with issues facing the general population and must attempt not only to balance a variety of health care needs, but to weigh them against other societal concerns.

Most health administrators neither provide direct patient care nor formulate public policy. Rather, they primarily influence allocation of resources in their own institutions. Here they are responsible for developing, implementing, and monitoring institutional policies and decisions to ensure that all patients, physicians, and employees are treated fairly.

Administrators are obligated to promote justice and act impartially, but there are so many competing principles and personal interests that they are often embroiled in dilemma and controversy. It is difficult to be fair in representing the interests of patients, owners or stockholders, third-party payers, and the community while at the same time keeping the hospital running smoothly and out of the red. Nonetheless, the principle of justice can provide a foundation, if not an easy solution, to the task.

Utility

The principle of utility dictates that "usefulness" or "balance" should be maintained in decision making; that is, one must balance the good and bad aspects of alternatives. Utility is often understood in terms of individual preference and selection of the act that creates the greatest good or the least harm for the greatest number.

For utilitarians the principle of utility is the single basic, most important ethical principle in guiding behavior. They argue that maximizing utility leads to the most desirable outcome. Others use the principle to balance the conflicts resulting from efforts to apply the first four principles. As such, utility becomes the one principle that bears more of a procedural than a substantive tone. Deontologists view utility less as a commanding procedural directive and more as a substantive objective worth seeking. Unlike most utilitarians, they would not necessarily give it priority over the other four principles.

Whatever the problem, it will be easier to analyze (and perhaps solve) if one takes ethical principles into account and uses them as a foundation for decision making.

References

Amundsen, Darrel. "History of medical ethics, medieval Europe: fourth to sixteenth century." In Warren T. Reich, ed., *The Encyclopedia of Bioethics*. New York: Free Press, 1978, pp. 938-951.

Austin, Charles J. "What is health administration?" *Hospital Administration* 19:14-29, Summer 1974.

Beauchamp, Tom L., and Norman E. Bowie. *Ethical Theory and Business*. 2nd edition. Englewood Cliffs, N.J.: Prentice-Hall, 1983.

Beauchamp, Tom L., and James F. Childress. *Principles of Biomedical Ethics*. 2nd edition. New York: Oxford University Press, 1983.

Beauchamp, Tom L., and Ruth R. Faden. "The right to health and the to right health care." *Journal of Medicine and Philosophy* 4(2):118-131, June 1979.

Beauchamp, Tom L., and Laurence B. McCullough. *Medical Ethics: The Moral Responsibilities of Physicians*. Englewood Cliffs, N.J.: Prentice-Hall, 1984.

Callahan, Daniel. "Applied ethics: a strategy for fostering professional responsibility." *Carnegie Quarterly* 28 (2-3):1-7, Spring/Summer 1980.

Childress, James F. "A right to health care." *Journal of Medicine and Philosophy* 4(2):132-147, June 1979.

Cunningham, Robert M. Jr. *The Healing Mission and the Business Ethic*. Chicago, Ill.: Pluribus Press, 1982.

Cunningham, Robert M. Jr. "More than a business: are hospitals forgetting their basic mission?" *Hospitals* 57:88-90, January 16, 1983.

DeGeorge, Richard T. "The moral responsibility of the hospital." *Journal of Medicine and Philosophy* 7(1): 87-100, February 1982.

Edelstein, Ludwig. "The Hippocratic Oath: text, translation, and interpretation." *Bulletin of the History of Medicine*, Supplement 1. Baltimore, Md.: Johns Hopkins University Press, 1943.

Fried, Charles. "Equality and rights in medical care." *Hastings Center Report* 6:29-34, February 1976.

Ginzberg, Eli. "The monitarization of medical care." *New England Journal of Medicine* 310(18):1162-1165, May 3, 1984.

Hiller, Marc D. "Ethics and health care administration: issues in education and practice." *Journal of Health Administration Education* 2(2):147-192, Spring 1984.

Kass, Leon J. "The new biology: what price relieving man's estate?" *Science* 174:779-788, 1971.

McGibony, John R. *Principles of Hospital Administration.* 2nd edition. New York: G. P. Putnam's Sons, 1969.

Mill, John Stuart, ed. *Utilitarianism, on Liberty, and Essay on Bentham.* New York: New American Library, 1974. (Originally published in 1861.)

Nozick, Robert. *Anarchy, State, and Utopia.* New York: Basic Books, 1974.

O'Rourke, Kevin. "An ethical perspective on investor-owned medical care corporations." *Frontiers of Health Services Management* 1(1):10-26, September 1984.

Outka, Gene. "Social justice and equal access to health care." *Journal of Religious Ethics* 2:11-32, 1974.

Pellegrino, Edmund D. "Medical morality and medical economics: the conflict of canons." *Hastings Center Report* 8:8-12, 1978.

Pellegrino, Edmund D. "Catholic hospitals: survival without moral compromise." *Health Progress* May 1985, pp. 42-49.

Pellegrino, Edmund D., and David C. Thomasma. *A Philosophical Basis of Medical Practice: Toward a Philosophy and Ethic of the Healing Professions.* New York: Oxford University Press, 1981.

Purtilo, Ruth B., and Christine K. Cassel. *Ethical Dimensions in the Health Professions.* Philadelphia, Pa.: W. B. Saunders Company, 1981.

33

Relman, Arnold S. "The new medical-industrial complex."
New England Journal of Medicine 303:963-970, October
23, 1980.

Relman, Arnold S. "Cost control, doctors' ethics, and
patient care." *Issues in Science and Technology* I:103-
111, Winter 1985.

Rosett, Richard N. "Doing well by doing good: investor-
owned hospitals." *Frontiers of Health Services Management* 1(1):2-9, September 1984.

Ross, William D. *The Right and the Good*. Oxford: Oxford
University Press, 1930.

Sade, Robert. "Medical care as a right: a refutation."
New England Journal of Medicine 285:1288-1292, December
2, 1971.

Sloan, Frank A., and Robert A. Vraciu. "Investor-owned
and not-for-profit hospitals: addressing some issues."
Health Affairs 2(1):25-37, Spring 1983.

Starkweather, David B. "In search of social enterprise:
a fable." *Hospital and Health Services Administration*
31(3):45-57, May/June 1986.

Starr, Paul. *The Social Transformation of American Medicine*. New York: Free Press, 1982.

Telfer, E. "Justice, welfare, and health care." *Journal
of Medical Ethics* 2:107-111, September 1976.

Veatch, Robert M. "What is a 'just' health care delivery?"
In Robert M. Veatch and Roy Branson, eds., *Ethics
and Health Policy*. Cambridge, Mass.: Ballinger Publishing Company, 1976.

Veatch, Robert M. "Just social institutions and the right
to health care." *Journal of Medicine and Philosophy*
4(2):170-173, June 1979.

Wikler, Daniel. "Forming an ethical response to for-profit health care." *Business and Health* 2(3):25-29, January/ February 1985.

Williams, David G. "Investor-owned versus not-for-profit hospitals: what are the issues?" *Frontiers of Health Services Management* 1(1):27-32, September 1984.

Young, Quentin D. "Impact of for-profit enterprise on health care." *Journal of Public Health Policy* 5(4): 449-452, 1984.

Young, Quentin D. "The danger of making serious problems worse." *Business and Health* 2(3):32-33, January/ February 1985.

CHAPTER 3

THE ETHICAL DIMENSION IN DECISION MAKING

In the past, health care was perceived as a moral right. But increasing costs of medical technology and the prolonging of life is forcing debate on the trade-off between the cost of medical care and the benefits that result. Yet unknown is whether a new social consensus will emerge on the priority of health care.

Health is now viewed as a social good as well as a commodity affected by political and economic forces. As Thurow (1984, p. 1572) asserts, "While health care costs are being treated as if they were largely an economic problem, they are not. To be solved, they will have to be treated as an ethical problem."

This is only one of many ethical issues that are forcing health administrators to confront a series of hard choices. McNerney (1985, p. 336) has argued that administrators must know what is going on in their institutions, be able to place ethical issues in perspective, and establish the necessary procedures to solve them. In addition to learning to make decisions, they must create opportunities for board and staff to appreciate and deal with a wide variety of ethical issues in a sensitive manner.

In addition to learning ethical theory and principles, administrators must be able to effectively apply ethics in their decision making. This paper discusses two different approaches for doing so.

WHAT CONSTITUTES ETHICAL PROBLEMS AND DILEMMAS?

First, an administrator must know when an ethical problem exists. Questions involving value judgments, as opposed to facts, do not necessarily precipitate ethical problems. Nevertheless, Simon (1945, p. 45) emphasizes that every decision involves both factual and value elements

37

and that both must be considered at all times. He argues that while factual propositions may be tested to determine whether they are absolute, the value component of administrative decisions is never fully reducible to factual terms that can be empirically confirmed.

In establishing the existence of an ethical problem, two components must be identified. First, a real choice must exist between possible courses of action. While many hypothetical situations can spring from efforts to solve an ethical dilemma, only *real* decision alternatives should be considered. However, all plausible-appearing alternatives should be included because it is important to identify *all* choices, regardless of their implications. Second, each possible action or its consequences must hold a significantly different value, and the administrator must be able to distinguish between ethics and values and to acknowledge that personal values often affect decisions.

Not all administrative problems constitute moral dilemmas; some are conflicts between an ethical obligation and self-interest or simply personal inclination. Thus, conflicts of interest do not pose truly ethical dilemmas. Furthermore, there is no ethical issue if potential choices or courses of action are unreal or impossible.

Ethical dilemmas exist when acting on the basis of one moral conviction means breaking another. In other words, when moral considerations (usually based on ethical principles) can be appealed to for each of two or more opposing courses of action, there is an ethical dilemma. These kinds of situations are common in health management. When they arise, the health care administrator must assess why and to what degree certain types of acts or character traits are morally "better" than others.

THE RELATIONSHIP BETWEEN LAW AND ETHICS

Sometimes when institutions or individuals fail to act, lawmakers (e.g., the courts, legislative bodies, executive orders) must intervene. Pellegrino and Thomasma (1981,

p. 247) contend that legal intervention marks "a forceful commentary on the tardiness" of institutions in meeting their ethical obligations. In supporting their claim, they refer to the "sharpening of the definitions of legal and fiscal accountability of boards and administrators for quality of care, protection of the rights of consent, managerial efficiency, equity in provision of services, and assuring rights of due process. Most of these obligations would have, and should have, been derived from a conscious reflection on the moral obligations implicit in what hospitals are about."

Increasingly, administrators have found themselves dealing with legal issues. Many have hired staff attorneys; most have at least placed legal counsel on retainer. Amid increasingly complex regulatory requirements and a highly litigious society, legal considerations have moved to the forefront of successful institutional management.

Many administrators erroneously assume that the law represents a codification of ethics and a means by which societal values are adjudicated. In other words, if something is legal, then it must also be ethical. This naive view has created a popular perception that simply obeying the law will also resolve ethical problems. Of course, there are issues on which law and ethics do coincide, and law has undeniably ensured certain rights and liberties, but there is often a large gap between what is legal and what is ethical; consider, for example, the issues of abortion and treatment of defective newborns. In both cases, the law has contradicted values strongly held by large segments of society, including those of some health care institutions and professionals.

Whereas law usually mandates minimum standards or criteria and enforces itself through sanctions and penalties, ethics tends to reach for the ideal. It is unbounded, voluntary, and cannot be mandated. Law is standardized, filled with procedural bureaucracy, and often impersonal. It fosters an adversarial process with a singular goal: winning. In contrast, ethics is more humanistic and personal and largely dependent on conscience. In most cases it is sensitive to the kinds of situations that arise in health care. Winning is not usually the issue, and choices are not as clear-cut. Rather, ethical analysis seeks to determine the "best" outcome from all possible alternatives.

Nonetheless, law and ethics can reinforce each other. Law protects against injustice and ensures rights, while ethics asks us to act on principles that often extend beyond the law. For example, the law provides for certain rights regarding informed consent and confidentiality, yet strict adherence to the principle of respect for persons may lead one to voluntarily extend beyond the intent of the law.

It is important to appreciate how the distinctions between law and ethics affect administration. Friedman and Friedman (1981) have described a simple hierarchical model of ethical behavior common to any profession or discipline. It is a four-tiered pyramid that illustrates how management is affected by whether practices are considered illegal or unethical. At the lowest level (level D) is illegal, high-risk behavior that most law-abiding business or health care managers would shun, such as price-fixing, embezzlement, and fraud, all of which carry legal sanctions. Level C contains illegal, low-risk activities, including failure to fully comply with affirmative action policies, applying for undeserved government support or subsidies, receiving kickbacks, or failing to fully inform patients of all risks and alternatives (informed consent) prior to surgery. All these activities are technically illegal but not uncommon, and only meticulously law-abiding people would reject them categorically. Level B includes behavior that is clearly unethical but not illegal, such as nepotism, "patient skimming," refusal to accept all patients in need, deceptive (but not false) advertising, or premature discharge practices based on DRG (diagnosis-related group) classification. While ethical administrators would not engage in such practices, these activities might meet varying degrees of acceptability by law-abiding unethical administrators. Level A consists of behavior that is certainly not illegal and that many would not consider unethical, such as promoting one's own hospital on its strength in a particular area while knowing that the closest competing hospital provides the same service, seeking to add a particular service that really is not truly needed solely to weaken competition, and offering services at an artificially low price to lure patients away from a competing institution and then suddenly raising the price. Level A acts must be carefully examined before being considered entirely ethical.

As in both law and ethics, the boundaries dividing levels D through A are often indistinct. Yet the model illustrates the relationship between illegal and unethical practices. Some of the examples reinforce the fact that not all problems of choice are ethical dilemmas; some are simply illegal.

Administrators often have to decide whether to take a stand on a principle for which there is no overwhelming prevailing legal counterpart, such as forgoing life-sustaining treatment. And some dilemmas that should remain private and to which only the people involved are privy are forced into painful, public adversarial proceedings because an administrator is justifiably fearful of potential institutional and professional liability risks.

LEVELS AT WHICH DILEMMAS OCCUR

Ethical issues related to health care in general and administration in particular arise at three levels: macro, meso, and micro. They occur when a sound ethical argument to do one thing conflicts with an equally sound argument to do another. While such conflicts frequently occur at a single level, further complexity arises when the basis of arguments is at different levels.

The macro level focuses on society or the community and often involves values reflected in social policies or governmental actions, such as access to medical care. This concern has resulted in legislation such as Medicaid and Medicare, spurred more than a half century of debate about national health insurance, and caused people to question whether health care ought to be a right or a privilege.

41

Macroallocation concerns have prompted health care institutions to respond to community-held values and needs, directly through establishing specific programs and indirectly through maintaining voluntary, community-oriented boards of directors (trustees).

Issues arising at the meso level focus on organizations and professions, and it is this level with which health administrators are primarily concerned. A classic dilemma here is the "cost-quality debate." Administrators are responsible for the survival of their institutions; thus circumstances may force them to sacrifice quality or cut back on services to save money. Competing with this managerial ethic of increased efficiency and cost containment are the traditional healing mission of health care professionals (Hiller, 1981) and the moral obligation of health care institutions to provide treatment (Cunningham, 1983).

Dilemmas arising at the micro, or individual, level are highly personal and frequently involve a physician-patient relationship or an issue of medical treatment. The classic issues encountered here are often referred to as "patient rights," in a moral rather than a legal sense. Inevitably, issues at this level are encountered personally by everyone during the course of a lifetime.

WHAT IS TO BE DECIDED AND WHO DECIDES?

Ethical questions are either substantive or procedural. Substantive questions involve morality and personal values. For example, how much free care should an institution provide, and how honest and principled do administrators have to be in an environment driven by competition? Procedural questions ask who should decide. Administrators may believe they should make all decisions by themselves (with input from the board), but they are often challenged by physicians, patients, communities, and even the courts. Classic procedural questions arise in trying to determine who should decide if and when life-support systems may be withdrawn from a patient, particularly when the patient lacks the capacity to express an opinion, or what person in need should be admitted to the last bed in an intensive care unit or receive the single available donor organ.

While both substantive and procedural questions create ethical dilemmas, all ethical principles can be applied to the former, whereas procedural dilemmas tend to emphasize conflicts of justice and/or respect for persons (i.e., personal liberty).

TYPES OF ETHICAL CONFLICT

Sometimes conflicts are a matter of conflicting principles, suggesting different outcomes. For example, respecting autonomy might not always be in one's best interest; in such a case, beneficence might take priority over autonomy. Other times, conflict arises from applying the same principle at different levels. For example, a situation may arise where what is best for a patient might not be in the institution's best interest, clearly posing a micromeso conflict.

While one must always use ethical principles to solve dilemmas, outcomes often reflect the way alternative choices are valued. Given the potential for personal values to influence decision making, administrators must periodically clarify their own values. They must also understand the independent ethical responsibilities of the institution in fulfilling its mission (Thomasma, 1982), for when personal values differ from the values of the institution or the profession, an uneasy situation exists at best.

In general, ethical conflicts fall into four broad categories which vary according to the values placed on the choices (Brody, 1981): (1) good versus evil, (2) better versus worse, (3) good versus good, and (4) allocation conflicts.

Conflicts Involving Good Versus Evil

The least troublesome ethical conflicts are those that involve choices clearly considered to be "good" or "evil." Administrators must be beware, however, of erroneously assuming that all ethical conflicts pose such genuinely clear-cut options: few do.

Conflicts Involving Better Versus Worse

In conflicts presenting choices that can be viewed only as "better" or "worse," decision making is not so simple. This is especially true when the units of value are different. For example, suppose an administrator is confronted with a dilemma about a question of fairness among employees. In analyzing the problem, the two best choices appear almost indistinguishable in terms of which is "better" or "worse." The first option will cost $20,000 and offer peace of mind; the second will cost $10,000 and involve considerable aggravation. Most ethical conflicts confronting administrators fall in this "better vs. worse" category.

Conflicts Involving Good Versus Good

In the third type of conflict situation, the administrator must choose between two mutually exclusive "goods" based on different motives and sound ethical principles. The problem is that each seemingly good action precludes another; thus one good alternative must be chosen over another even though both are based on good motives and sound ethical principles. Inevitably, the selection process dictates a prioritization of principles. Regardless of the decision, the outcome will often be perceived as "bad" by some because people tend to view the failure to do good as bad. For example, suppose an administrator has to make a decision about forgoing life-sustaining treatment for a suffering, terminally ill patient in an institution that has no formal policy on this issue. Assume that the patient, his family, and his physicians all agree that no

44

further action should be taken to sustain life. To continue life support would mean greater pain and suffering, contradict the patient's wish to be allowed to die with dignity, and violate the principle of respect for persons.

The administrator understands that compliance with the patient's request ensures the individual's autonomy, but doing so would deny a second, equally compelling good. The institution has a moral obligation to prolong life, and to cut off life could be viewed as harming the patient (violating the principle of nonmaleficence) and possibly put the institution in legal jeopardy. It might also risk violating the community's trust, something not to be taken lightly given the institution's dependence on community support.

Another potential "good versus good conflict" might involve caring for severely defective newborns. In this situation, which is highly controversial, the government has imposed regulations that require hospitals to treat these infants. For administrators whose institutions provide neonatal care, there are two choices: deciding not to treat the infant because that is the parents' wish (and the doctors agree) or deciding to save (or simply extend) the infant's life. The decision requires choosing one of two mutually exclusive goods. This problem illustrates complications that can arise when law invades the realm of ethical decision making. In such a case, many administrators might be tempted to choose a "legal" good out of fear of a potential lawsuit.

As an actual example of the conflict that can arise between law and ethics, take the case of *Grizwold versus Connecticut*. In 1965, physicians knowingly violated an antiquated law by giving contraceptive information to an unmarried woman. This led to a landmark U.S. Supreme Court decision that overturned the Connecticut law between law and ethics (Ladd, 1979).

Abortion is another example. If an institution upholds a pregnant woman's right to privacy by giving her freedom of choice, it is showing respect for persons. But, if it refused her an abortion, it would be preserving the sanctity of life, another good. To date, both the courts and legislatures have been unsuccessful in their attempts to resolve this conflict between the two mutually exclusive goods.

Another common conflict has to do with respect for confidentiality of patient information, which health care institutions and physicians are ethically bound to uphold. However, people outside the institution sometimes have valid reasons for wanting access to such information. A conflict between two goods then arises, as, for example, when public health or safety is involved in controlling the spread of communicable diseases, in restraining persons who might be dangerous to others, or in releasing patient data to third parties such as Blue Cross, Medicaid, or Medicare. The institution is in the middle and must decide whether to risk a demise of the physician-patient relationship (Hiller and Seidel, 1982).

All this puts administrators in a moral bind, and no matter what they choose, they are still in an uncomfortable position because many people believe that failure to act on one good choice means that the alternative is somehow "bad." Such conflicts are particularly thorny because administrators feel they always have to second-guess their decisions.

Conflicts Involving Allocation

Brody (1981, p. 9) has dubbed allocation conflicts as "the principle of 'you can't have your cake and eat it too.'" Here, choosing one course of action constitutes a decision not to choose others and thus reflects a value judgment. Most such conflicts involve rationing scarce resources such as money or time. In an era of competition and tight finances, administrators must often support one project, department, or demand over others. In doing so, they allocate a resource for one thing while simultaneously withholding it from something else. Such decisions typically reflect an adherence to one or more material principles of justice over others.

These four general types of ethical conflict (good and evil, better and worse, two mutually exclusive goods, and allocation) represent a basic classification scheme. Because ethical problems can be so variable and highly complicated, there is an infinite number of potential conflict types. This necessitates that great importance be placed on the process by which such dilemmas are analyzed, the subject of the following section.

RESOLVING ETHICAL DILEMMAS

Many problems confronting administrators require a process of ethical analysis or decision making. Undertaking such a procedure is described by Pellegrino as "doing ethics." Administrators who recognize their career as decision makers may look askance at this statement and ask what is so different about ethical decision making from other types of decision making. Does it lie in the methods of decision making? In the conclusions reached? In the assumptions used? In all or none of these? (Hill et al., 1978, p. 36).

That which is distinctive about doing ethics rests in the centrality of fundamental ethical principles, both in the reasoning that leads up to the decision and in that the decision maker accepts the principle in question as part of his or her value orientation. (The latter requires a prior clarification of values, often done using structured exercises.)

An administrator "makes an ethical decision, as distinct from some other kind of decision, if and only if he decides what to do by essential reliance upon some ethical rule, principle, standard, or norm" (Hill et al., 1978, p. 36). This means that if an administrator did not rely on an ethical principle in reaching a decision, then the decision he made may not be the same one he would have reached had he applied ethics or, had the same decision been made, the reason behind it would have differed and not been based on an ethical principle. Rather, it would have had another basis, such as profitability, business efficiency, or even self-interest.

While ethical decision making focuses on principles and values, it is essential to realize two basic points. First, in addition to the five fundamental principles already described, there are others. Moreover, the hierarchy of moral justification provided by Beauchamp and Childress (1983, p. 5) and highlighted in the previous chapter illustrates the general and fundamental nature of principles from which a larger number of more specific "rules" are derived. Second, since the class of principles does not always lead to resolution, it is valuable to move the analysis to a theoretical level, that which Beauchamp and Childress describe as the most general. By referring occasionally to major theories, one can often resolve conflict between principles and rules.

The remainder of this chapter focuses on providing administrators with two useful, albeit different, ways to analyze ethical dilemmas. The use of such techniques, regardless of the type of ethical conflict, will strengthen the ability of administrators to analyze and justify their decisions to themselves, their institutions and employees, and their communities.

While multiple approaches toward ethical decision making have been developed (Hill et al., 1978; Purtilo and Cassel, 1981, pp. 27-29; Brody, 1981, pp. 9-15, 353-357; Harron, Burnside, and Beauchamp, 1983, pp. 4-5), none guarantees resolution of all quandaries. Essential to all, however, is the recognition of basic ethical principles from which institutional policies and administrative decisions should be derived. Furthermore, each attempts to ensure a systematic examination of alternative courses of action based on comprehending fundamental ethical principles and appreciating personal, institutional, and societal values.

48

The first of the two approaches presented here reflects a qualitative orientation commonly used in ethical decision making in medicine; the second emphasizes a mathematical framework and is strongly grounded in quantitative techniques more often employed in business management. Both approaches reflect the centrality of fundamental ethical principles being used to resolve ethical problems.

Prior to undertaking either approach, administrators must realize that outcomes (i.e., decisions or actions) often vary as a result of what level (i.e., community, institutional, or individual) is given priority during decision making. However, neither approach intrinsically facilitates a consideration of level. Administrators must acknowledge the potential competition among levels and determine the level at which the analysis is to be conducted. Any effort to justify a final decision in a situation in which a multilevel conflict exists, such as whether the decision will be more beneficial to the community or to the institution, can be strengthened by conducting similar analyses from the perspective of each level. If the respective ethical outcomes differ, the decision maker is able to consciously accept one over the other knowing that both were ethically justifiable but that the final decision gave priority to one level over another.

Qualitative Approach

The qualitative approach consists of a six-step process outlined by Harron, Burnside, and Beauchamp (1983, pp. 4-5) that considers each of the critical elements needed to make an ethically sound decision. It maximizes a rational systematic examination of alternative courses of action based on the application of fundamental ethical principles. The most successful use of this process requires that administrators have clarified their personal values. While personal and professional values will affect ultimate decisions, their influence should be limited (see Step 5).

Step 1. Identifying the Problem

Identification represents three activities: perception, identification, and confirmation of an ethical problem. For an ethical problem to exist, there must be a real choice between possible courses of action, and one must place a significantly different value on each possible outcome. While such efforts are necessary, they are not wholly sufficient since not all problems truly constitute ethical dilemmas. For example, situations that pit acting in an ethical manner against acting in self-interest do not pose ethical problems. Furthermore, because many ethical dilemmas defy legal solutions (e.g., laws or policies governing abortion, forgoing life-sustaining treatments), seeking or obtaining legal resolutions or actions does not necessarily guarantee ethical solutions.

Step 2. Analysis of Alternatives

This step calls for administrators to list all alternative courses of action that could be used to address a problem. Usually, consideration of decision alternatives does not produce an exhaustive list; rather, only two options are considered—for example, to do or not to do something.

Human conditioning prefers seeing only two alternatives: it is easier to think in terms of "either-or" than to struggle with several alternatives that require some form of matrix-like analysis. Unfortunately, there are usually more than two alternatives to ethical problems, and thus it is essential to delineate all possible alternatives, even those that may appear somewhat remote.

In considering alternatives, administrators should not immediately discard those that initially appear to be in the best interests of others such as staff members, patients, or the community.

Step 3. Weighing Competing Options

This step requires that the consequences of each possible option be considered and then the most likely results assessed. The most dramatic consequences are immediately obvious, but there are usually more obscure ones as well. Sometimes they are interrelated or aggregated and have both short- and long-term impacts. They can affect a community, an institution or department, an individual, or a combination of all three, in which case yet another conflict may be created.

Some consequences are more important than others and must be balanced against each other. Not all are predictable, and administrators must realize that things may not turn out as they had thought. Often this is the stage where the varying importance of particular alternatives may be observed as a function of the level from which the analysis is being conducted. When this is the case, administrators need to acknowledge their frame of reference.

While it is common to think of individual or independent consequences, the degree to which effects may be interrelated or aggregated must be assessed as well. Sometimes, resolving conflicting alternatives and consequences requires minimal compromise; at other times, considerable sacrifice is required at one level or by one party.

Among the most difficult realities to be reckoned with is that the process of weighing options commonly generates a degree of uncertainty, given the impossibility of being able to predict every possible consequence for every alternative. Hence, at some point, the weighing process must give way to justification.

Step 4. Justification by Principle

Justification means the application of relevant principles or rules to alternatives and their consequences in a process through which one joins a good and sufficient moral reason for an action, based on an ethical principle or rule, to an alternative. This can mean attaching priority to highly valued ethical principles. Competing alternatives need to be examined critically in terms of their respective ability to withstand serious ethical inquiry.

For example, assume a choice rests between ensuring someone's right to privacy, based on the principle of autonomy, and guaranteeing fairness, based on the principle of justice. The choice depends on which principle is valued over the other *in this instance*.

Step 5. Making a Choice

At this point, the administrator selects an alternative based on a justifiable argument. However, many ethical dilemmas that require administrative decisions demand choosing from more than a single "good" alternative. Legitimate grounds often exist for selecting multiple alternatives based on different ethical principles. Hence, initial choices frequently reflect how the principles were prioritized in Step 4 and therefore may not meet with unanimous agreement.

Inevitably, some, if not most, choices mirror professional and personal value judgments. While the process has avoided their formal consideration to this point, it is only reasonable that they be acknowledged here. Assuming that administrators have consciously and sufficiently clarified their values, including moral teachings, these values may at this point bear some influence on the pending choices. Moreover, administrators must ascertain, control, and defend the extent to which they allow their values to affect their decision making. To the extent that personal values conflict with prior ethical deliberations, further wrestling with the problem at hand may be in order before a choice is made.

Step 6. Reassessing Choices

Administrators must now reexamine their choices and the justification for them, determine whether any unresolved questions remain, and relate the choice made to similar cases (elsewhere and at other times). While this step

tends to be the most often neglected in the haste to reach
a conclusion, such retrospective analysis should be made
before taking action based on the decision.

In comparing the current problem to similar ones,
things can be found that warrant reconsideration. This
may be characterized as a sort of "ethical safety net"
in that it assures that before making what may be an irrev-
ocable decision (or implementing an action based on one),
the decision maker is able to firmly support and justify
the decision on sound ethical grounds. Thomasma (1978)
suggests that it may be useful to think of criticisms that
could be lodged against the choice and come up with ways
to logically defend it.

A Quantitative Approach ✳

Given the many possible options frequently encountered
in making difficult ethical decisions, some have suggested
a more structured empirical approach that permits mathematical analysis (Hill et al., 1978; Francoeur, 1983).
The steps in this approach actually bear many of the same
qualitative judgments as those in the first approach; thus,
while the methodology reflects many elements similar to
those used in quantitative decision making, such as as-
signing numerical values to selection criteria and queuing
various alternatives (i.e., the construction of a decision
matrix), it still remains more qualitative (value-oriented)
than absolute (fact-oriented).

It may be argued that to the extent that a quantitative
methodology is used to make ethical decisions, sensitivity
is sacrificed. Whether quantitative decision making theory
can be used in resolving ethical dilemmas bears individual
scrutiny. If used, however, the decision matrix technique
is more structured and detailed and may serve as a rational
mechanism for examining a large range of administrative
alternatives. Furthermore, its efficiency increases as
the number of alternatives increases (Hill et al., 1978,
p. 120). As a decision aid, it forces a detailed analysis
of each option in light of the imposed ethical criteria

and the weights given to these criteria based on personal
and professional values.

To illustrate the application of this approach, let
us look at an example of a common ethical dilemma confronting health care institutions: *Should a community hospital
deny care to the indigent or the uninsured?*

Step 1. Identifying Alternatives

The initial step in using a decision matrix is to
identify all possible ethically justifiable alternatives.
No feasible option should be included, since this structured
approach does not facilitate later additions or modifica-
tions.   The effectiveness of the analysis is a function
of the number of alternatives included in the matrix.
Upon identification, each alternative should be listed.

In the case study, the administrator of Community
Hospital would initially identify the alternatives that
are ethically acceptable.   (Since the example is being
used for demonstration purposes, our concern here rests
with illustrating the process rather than seeking a single
"best" outcome.) Only three alternative policies are considered for Community Hospital. If this were an actual
case in which the outcome was critical, more effort would
be undertaken to generate potentially relevant alternatives
to maximize the effectiveness of this analytical process.

Alternative 1: Hospital care should be denied
to individuals unable to pay.

Alternative 2: Hospital care should be provided
only to a limited number of individuals unable
to pay (not to exceed 8 percent of net annual
revenues).

Alternative 3: Hospital care should not be denied
to any individual based solely on his or her
inability to pay. (This is Community Hospitals's
present policy and as such should always be considered as an alternative.)

54

Step 2. Determining the Evaluation Criteria

The second step of the quantitative approach requires identification of those criteria (ethical principles, rules, and other selected factors) to be used in evaluating each alternative generated in Step 1. Since the objective is to determine the options based on fundamental ethical principles and rules, the following seven criteria are commonly used in deriving value statements:

1. **Beneficence**--contributing to the good and welfare of others;
2. **Nonmaleficence**--doing no harm to others;
3. **Truth-telling**--being honest with others;
4. **Confidentiality**--guarding against the dissemination of private personal information;
5. **Autonomy (self-determination)**--ensuring the freedom of individuals to make their own decisions in the absence of coercion;
6. **Justice**--ensuring fairness and equality in decisions concerning individuals;
7. **Utility**--balancing the above criteria in a manner that promises the best overall outcome in each situation.

In addition to the above list of ethical criteria, other factors that reflect little if any ethical content (e.g., economic, political, legal, or philosophical concerns) may be added selectively to avoid risking undue criticism. However, they should be allocated low weights in the matrix.

The administrator must determine which of the above criteria are applicable in light of the specific ethical problem at hand. While any two administrators applying these criteria to a particular ethical problem may reach different conclusions, there should be little question as to the applicability of the criteria.

Step 3. Deriving "Value Statements" from Criteria

From the criteria identified in Step 2, "value statements" relevant to an ethical dilemma may be developed. Using the sample case, eight criteria were deemed relevant: beneficence, nonmaleficence, autonomy, justice, and utility, as well as certain philosophical, political, and legal factors. (The value statements derived from these criteria are not meant to be exhaustive.)

Under the principle of beneficence, two value statements were identified: the hospital should provide care to patients who need it, and others should be treated as we would like to be treated. Under nonmaleficence, a third value statement was developed: the hospital should never deny care to an individual when doing so may result in (further) harm. Under autonomy: individuals have a moral claim, or right, to health care when they are sick. This value statement may gain more validity when an institution receives benefits such as tax-free status or large public subsidies.

Some ethical dilemmas arise due to competing interests and limited resources. For example, that which may be in the best interest of an institution may not serve the best interests of individual patients or the community. Not surprisingly, the principle of justice usually precipitates several value statements based on one or more material principles. In this case, only two statements are identified, although others could be expressed: a hospital should promote an equitable distribution of limited resources, and ensuring unlimited care to everyone would result in care being available to no one (i.e., the hospital could not survive financially).

The principle of utility generates a seventh statement: the hospital should promote maximum community health. In employing such a principle, Community Hospital would commit itself to using its resources in a manner that benefits the greatest number (recognizing that in doing so, some may be harmed).

Three "nonethical" criteria that may be given administrative consideration were identified. The philosophical criterion concerns the existing institutional mission: the hospital will serve all who enter it in need of medical care. Political sensitivity leads to a ninth criterion: the hospital should maintain a positive community image. This statement illustrates the importance of public support and maintaining positive community esteem.

Step 4. Rank Ordering and Calculating Weighting Factors for Value Statements

The next step in formulating the matrix analysis requires that weights be determined for each value statement by rank ordering the statements in order of perceived importance.

As illustrated in Table 3, the most important statement is listed first and assigned a 10; the least important is assigned a 1. Should two or more value statements be viewed equally important, they may be clustered together, in which case they will have the same rank order.

After the value statements have been ordered, the "weighting factor" is calculated for each statement in a two-part process: (1) summation of the numbers in the ordering column (in this example, the total is 55) and (2) division of the order of each value statement by the total. Any value statements assigned the same order would clearly have equal weighting factors.

Step 5. Rating the Alternatives

In constructing the decision matrix (see Table 4), the alternatives are listed on the left-hand side of the table. The value statements are listed down the side of the matrix, starting with the highest value on the left and ending with the lowest value. Then the weighting factor for each value statement is inserted into the matrix.

Next, each alternative is rated on a scale of 10 (highest) to 1 (lowest). This rating reveals the degree to

TABLE 3   Ordering and Weighting Value Statements for Community Hospital

Value Statement	Order	Weighting Factor (order/total order)
The hospital should promote maximum community health.	10	0.18
Ensuring unlimited care to everyone would result in care being available to no one.	9	0.16
The hospital should never deny care to an individual when doing so may result in harm to the individual.	8	0.15
Others should be treated as we would like to be treated.	7	0.13
The hospital should provide care to all patients needing it.	6	0.11
The hospital should promote the equitable distribution of limited resources.	5	0.09
The hospital is legally required to provide emergency room care to stabilize a patient's condition.	4	0.07
Individuals have a right to care when they are sick.	3	0.05
The hospital should maintain a positive image in the community to sustain its continued support.	2	0.04
The hospital will serve all who enter it in need of medical care.	1	0.02
Total	55	1.00

Table 4   Constructing a Decision Matrix: A Sample Case Study

Alternative 1: Hospital care should be denied to individuals unable to pay.

Alternative 2: Hospital care should be provided only to a limited number of individuals unable to pay (not to exceed 8 percent of net annual revenues).

Alternative 3: Hospital care should not be denied to any individual based solely on their inability to pay. (This is Community Hospitals's present policy and as such should always be considered as an alternative.)

VALUES	ORDER	WEIGHT	ALT 1	ALT 2	ALT 3
The hospital should promote maximum community health.	10	0.18	1	4	10
			0.18	0.72	1.80
Ensuring unlimited care to everyone would result in care being available to no one.	9	0.16	10	6	3
			1.60	0.96	0.48
The hospital must never deny care to an individual if doing so may result in harm to the individual.	8	0.15	1	5	8
			0.15	0.75	1.20
Others should be treated as we would like to be treated.	7	0.13	2	4	10
			0.26	0.52	1.30
The hospital should provide care to all patients needing it.	6	0.11	1	4	10
			0.11	0.44	1.10
The hospital should promote the equitable distribution of limite resources.	5	0.09	1	7	7
			0.09	0.63	0.63
The hospital is required to provide emergency room care to stabilize a patient's condition.	4	0.07	2	4	10
			0.14	0.28	0.70
Individuals have a right to care when they are sick.	3	0.05	1	3	8
			0.05	0.15	0.40
The hospital should maintain a positive image in the community to sustain its continued support.	2	0.04	2	4	10
			0.08	0.16	0.40
The hospital will serve all who enter it in need of medical care	1	0.02	1	4	10
			0.02	0.08	0.20
TOTAL	55	1.00	2.68	4.69	8.21

Format from Hill et al., 1978, pp. 124-126.

to which the administrator believes that selecting each of the possible alternatives would achieve or promote a particular value. This numerical rating is referred to as a rating factor. For example, each of the three alternatives previously identified for Community Hospital is rated on the 10 to 1 scale with respect to its achieving or promoting each of the values (as expressed by the value statements). Using each value statement, each alternative is successively rated.

More specifically, the decision matrix indicates the extent (10 = most; 1 = least) to which the first value promoting maximum community health would be achieved or promoted by choosing the first alternative (denying health care to those unable to pay), the second alternative (providing a limited amount of free care), the third alternative (not denying care to anyone due to an inability to pay), and so on. These respective rating factors are then inserted in the upper half (above the diagonal line) of each square making up the body of the matrix. Rating factors are determined one at a time, value by value, until each cell has been filled.

Step 6. Completing the Matrix and Making the Decision

To complete the decision matrix, the appropriate weighting factor from each row is multiplied by each rating factor recorded in the upper half of each cell. The product is then recorded in the lower half of the cell (below the diagonal line). This is done until each cell is filled with a rating factor and a product of the rating and weighting factors.

Then, all the products for each column are added, and the sum is entered in the "total" row under the appropriate alternative. Since all weighting factors must total 1.0 and the highest rating factor is 10, a perfect sum (i.e., maximum score) would be 10 (or 100 percent if percentages are preferred).

Finally, the level of confidence is determined for each possible alternative by reviewing the sum column.

The alternative with the highest ranking should be the most ethical of all those considered.

Use of the decision matrix in ethical decision making has the advantage of providing administrators with the ability to clearly present and document their decisions to other parties. Furthermore, it affords an opportunity to carefully reassess or reaffirm the decision making process, and potentially its outcome. The effective use of this technique, however, demands total honesty and thoroughness by those attempting to resolve difficult ethical dilemmas. While the approach bears a quantitative orientation, many of the variables assigned by decision makers are based on qualitative judgments. Hence, less than honest administrators may not only fool themselves in erroneously justifying a particular decision, but may also arrive at a decision that manipulates the technique to justify a predetermined goal (Hill et al., 1978, p. 127).

Given a meaningful appreciation of fundamental ethical principles and the ability to use them in critical decision making situations, health administrators can be better prepared to meet their growing institutional and professional challenges. Skill and expertise in conducting ethical analyses, particularly amid the thorny dilemmas posed by the plethora of choices inherent in administrative decision making, is an essential professional responsibility. Being able to justify decisions on solid ethical grounds contributes to an improved sense of both professional and personal competency. And the application of a generic set of ethical principles permits sound decision making without having to depend on a more limited, often too restrictive and specific code of ethics, regardless of the approach adopted.

References

Beauchamp, Tom L., and James F. Childress. *Principles of Biomedical Ethics*. 2nd edition. New York: Oxford University Press, 1983.

Brody, Howard. *Ethical Decisions in Medicine*. 2nd edition. Boston, Mass.: Little, Brown and Company, 1981.

Cunningham, Robert M. Jr. "More than a business: are hospitals forgetting their basic mission?" *Hospitals* 57:88-90, January 16, 1983.

Francoeur, Robert T. *Biomedical Ethics: A Guide to Decisionmaking*. New York: John Wiley & Sons, Inc., 1983.

Friedman, Hershey H., and Linda W. Friedman. "Ethics: everybody's business." *Collegiate News and Views*, Winter 1981-1982, pp. 11-13.

Harron, Frank, John Burnside, and Tom Beauchamp. *Health and Human Values: A Guide to Making Your Own Decisions*. New Haven, Conn.: Yale University Press, 1983.

Hill, Percy H., et al. *Making Decisions: A Multidisciplinary Introduction*. Reading, Mass.: Addison-Wesley Publishing Company, Inc., 1978.

Hiller, Marc D. "Medical ethics and public policy." In Marc D. Hiller, ed. *Medical Ethics and The Law: Implications for Public Policy*. Cambridge, Mass.: Ballinger Publishing Company, 1981, pp. 3-45.

Hiller, Marc D., and Lee F. Seidel. "Patient care management systems, medical records, and privacy." *Public Health Reports* 97(4):332-344, July-August, 1982.

Ladd, John. "Legalism and medical ethics." *Journal of Medicine and Philosophy* 4:70-71, 1979.

McNerney, Walter C. "Managing ethical dilemmas." *Journal of Health Administration Education* 3(3):331-340, Summer 1985.

Pellegrino, Edmund D., and David C. Thomasma. *A Philosophical Basis of Medical Practice: Toward a Philosophy and Ethic of the Healing Professions*. New York: Oxford University Press, 1981.

Purtilo, Ruth B., and Christine K. Cassel. *Ethical Dimensions in the Health Professions*. Philadelphia, Pa.: W. B. Saunders Company, 1981.

Simon, Herbert A. *Administrative Behavior: A Study of Decisionmaking in Administrative Organizations*. New York: Free Press, 1945.

Thomasma, David C. "Training in medical ethics: an ethical workup." *Forum in Medicine* December 1978, pp. 33-36.

Thomasma, David C. "Hospitals' ethical responsibilities as technology, regulation grow." *Hospital Progress* 63:74-79, December 1982.

Thurow, Lester Carl. "Learning to say 'no.'" *New England Journal of Medicine* 311(24):1569-1572, December 13, 1984.

Sellit, Claude S., and Marie C. Thomsen. Perform complications after anesthesia. Medical Journal. Guidelines on the Reading. Philadelphia: W. B. Saunders Company, 1980.

Robins, Frank. Pharmacologics & Cases. Historical signs in the Texas Examination. Philadelphia: W. B. Saunders Company, 1981.

Simon, Herbert A. Administrative Behavior, A study of Decision-Making Processes in Organizations. New York: Free Press, 1947.

Rosenberg, M. "On Standards of a medical Professional Values in Practice." December, 18 pp., 20-28.

Thomas, Harold G. "Residual educational responsibility, the professional regulation program." Medical Progress, March, 3:2-14, 1966.

Taylor, Lester Carl. "Leader, leadership, Handbook." Journal of Education Administration, Bibliography, 13. December. . . . .

CHAPTER 4

ETHICAL ISSUES CONFRONTING HEALTH ADMINISTRATION

On behalf of the medical staff, the chief of medicine asks the CEO to launch a new heart transplant program. The CEO knows that such a program will mean eliminating several primary care programs designed to improve community health.

A group of nurses and laboratory workers have prepared a statement about caring for AIDS patients. They submit it to the administrator and ask him to create a hospital policy that will permit them to refuse to care for AIDS victims.

A neurosurgeon at a tertiary care institution refuses to admit a transfer patient with severe head trauma when he learns that she has no insurance. This physician had previously been reprimanded by hospital administration for admitting another critically ill, uninsured patient. (Wrenn, 1985, p. 373)

A high school senior is admitted to a community hospital with evidence of spinal cord injury after an automobile accident. When it becomes apparent that he will be a quadriplegic, the youngster asks that all medical treatment, food, and water be discontinued. His physicians reject his plea for what they consider "hospital assisted" suicide. The case is brought to the CEO for action.

While most health administration problems involving ethical issues are not as dramatic as these, such cases illustrate the need to know how to resolve ethical dilemmas.

Treatment options never imagined a decade ago are now commonplace, including the prolonging of life beyond "natural" limits. High technology is expensive and creates conflict arising from changing economic conditions and competition. Indeed, health care is now an economic as well as a social good (Reinhardt, 1985). Furthermore, the public knows more about and expects more from hospitals and other health care organizations. It is willing to debate public policy issues and question the accessibility and quality of care.

While administrators need not become ethicists, they are increasingly being forced to wrestle with ethical dilemmas. This creates two important obligations: (1) administrators must recognize the existence of ethical issues, and (2) they must apply fundamental ethical theories and principles to decision making. In other words, they must understand what constitutes an ethical problem and how to use ethical principles to resolve that problem.

Attempts to classify ethical problems are not new, but past efforts have been somewhat premature or incomplete. It would be desirable to develop a simple matrix into which each type of ethical problem would fall, but this is easier said than done, given the brief history of the profession of health administration and the proliferation of complex issues to which its members must respond. There are, however, a variety of approaches that may be taken in examining ethical problems, although none appears fully satisfactory. Grouping the types of conflicts inherent in the profession seems to provide a reasonable, pragmatic, and workable approach. Such a tactic should focus on the degree to which competing interests force administrators to deviate from the historical healing mission of health organizations and the health professions. This is known as the competing interest accountability model and is discussed in detail below. First, however, let us review several other approaches for comparison.

THE MICRO-MESO-MACRO LEVEL APPROACH

As illustrated in previous works (Hiller, 1981, 1984), ethical issues can be discussed at three general levels: micro, macro, and meso.

The Micro Level

The micro level of discussion involves questions or relationships among individuals. It focuses on personal and professional guides to individual action or conduct. Issues at this level also involve professional relationships, such as those between physician and patient or administrator and staff member, and the conflicts that arise when personal values do not coincide with professional ones. Such conflicts may occur between individuals with different values or even within one individual whose personal and professional values conflict. For example, the issue of information disclosure often precipitates ethical conflict because people have different views about the value of confidentiality and privacy. Moreover, one's personal values on this subject (e.g., to maintain total confidentiality) may clash with one's professional obligation (e.g., to release certain confidential data to various agencies to ensure financial reimbursement for services rendered to a patient).

The Macro Level

Here, issues generally affect large numbers of people or certain population groups and tend to reflect certain social and/or cultural values, norms, or standards. When government policies and judicial decisions try to resolve ethical dilemmas, it is at the macro level. For example, the issue of whether the poor have a right to equal access to medical care would most likely be debated at the societal level. From a macro perspective, individual privacy would justifiably be sacrificed if necessary to ensure controlling the spread of a communicable disease.

The Meso Level

The most complex and least examined of the three levels is the meso (Hiller 1984), which exists between the micro and macro levels and at times overlaps them. This level is of primary concern to health administrators and board directors (trustees) because they must confront a variety of ethical dilemmas in establishing, implementing, and enforcing institutional policies. Also at the meso level is the conflict between administrative ethics--those of the profession of health administration--and organizational (institutional) ethics--representing the mission (corporate philosophy) of the institution.

Identifying or categorizing ethical problems by "level" has both advantages and disadvantages. Although most ethical issues can be grouped on such a basis, having only three levels may not provide sufficient distinctions for certain issues; and some particularly complex dilemmas do not fit neatly into any one level. Thus, from an analytical point of view, it may be useless to place a dilemma into a specific level; and furthermore, attempts to do so may prove somewhat arbitrary or reflect personal values or bias.

THE ETHICAL CODE APPROACH

Codes of ethics provide another approach to examining ethics in health administration.

Professional Codes of Ethics

The collective posture of a profession emerges at the meso, or institutional level and is stated in its code of ethics, which defines and guides acceptable and unacceptable conduct. Most health professions have a code of ethics; in fact, most believe it is a fundamental attribute of a profession (Greenwood, 1957). Conflict often arises, however, when a code is unclear about the difference between professional ethics and responsibilities and personal ethics and values. For example, how far do the demands of one's profession extend before they collide with one's personal values? Health administrators face this kind of conflict constantly.

While professional codes vary considerably, most are either so general and vague that they preclude enforcement, or so specific and practice-oriented that they offer little guidance in problem solving or decision making. The most useful and meaningful codes have a theoretical orientation based on ethical principles rather than a detailed recitation of do's and don't's, which has limited usefulness and generally provides "far too blunt an instrument for the fine work of decision-making" (Levey and Hill, 1986).

Possibly the best known and most respected contemporary code, revised several times since it was first written in 1847, is the "Principles of Medical Ethics" of the American Medical Association (Beauchamp and McCullough, 1984, p. 7). The most recent version, adopted in 1980, suggests a trend toward increasing generality of principles, a loosening of specific prohibitions, and an increasing recognition of patients' rights (Veatch, 1983). Historical documents such as the Hippocratic writings (fifth to fourth centuries B.C.) and Percival's "Medical Ethics" (1803) must also be acknowledged.

Ethical Codes in Health Administration

The American College of Healthcare Executives (ACHE) and the American Hospital Association (AHA) have both provided leadership in codes of ethics in health administration.

The ACHE, founded in 1933 and known as the American College of Hospital Administrators until 1985, is a major professional association of health care administrators. The AHA represents the nation's largest trade association comprised of health care institutions and has many affiliated groups of health professionals. In 1939 the two groups collaborated on a joint Code of Ethics (Neuhauser,

1983), which sets forth the fundamental ethical mission governing health care institutions. In it, they made a comprehensive statement about the central values of a hospital and of health care in general:

> The hospital is to render care to the sick and injured as its primary responsibility. Financial concerns and other interests should be of secondary consideration. The duty of the hospital is also to advance scientific knowledge and education of all participating in the work, and to take an active part in the promotion of general health. (AHA and ACHA, 1941)

The proclamation was modified in 1947, 1957, and 1963. The 1957 revision produced the following:

> Recognizing that the care of the sick is their first responsibility and a sacred trust, hospitals must at all times strive to provide the best possible care and treatment to all in need of health care. Such institutions, cognizant of their unique role of safeguarding the nation's health, should seek through compassionate and scientific care and health education to extend life, alleviate suffering, and improve the general health of the community they serve. (AHA and ACHA, 1957)

Eventually, conflicts arose between the members of the two groups, and in 1967, they reverted back to separate codes. Many of the conflicts precipitating the split appeared to result from changing environmental conditions, including increasing competition and the profit motive in health care. Neuhauser (1983) suggests that one reason for the separation was the AHA's reluctance to impose sanctions on member institutions that violated the Code.

In 1967 the AHA adopted its Guidelines on Ethical Conduct and Relationships for Health Care Institutions (see Appendix A). It was further revised in 1974 and 1980.

70

Responding to the growing competition in the hospital industry, the 1980 revision included an allowance for institutional marketing of services and soliciting of new patients (Neuhauser, 1983, p. 76). These and other changes marked an increasing AHA awareness of institutional financial concerns.

In 1973, the ACHA developed its Code of Ethics (see Appendix B), which included provisions about administrators' accountability to the College for their actions as institutional executives. It, too, was revised in 1973 and 1980, and at present is undergoing extensive review. While ACHA members are bound to the Code, they are also expected to adhere to the AHA's Guidelines for health care institutions, thus creating a dual accountability—to their profession and to their institution. As stated in The Preamble of the 1980 ACHA Code of Ethics:

> The ACHA Code of Ethics is specifically designed to define and set forth broad guidelines applicable to the personal (professional) accountability of all members of top-level management involved in the administration of hospitals, other health institutions, and related health activities represented in the mix of its membership. It is united in purpose with the Code of Ethics of the American Hospital Association, which defines standards of conduct for health institutions.

While there are natural linkages between the ACHA and AHA codes, these codes do represent different organizations. The ACHA is the organization to which individual health administrators are ethically bound, regardless of their employer. Thus, at least in theory, the ACHA Code could have a more far-reaching effect than the AHA's. But since many hospitals, particularly investor-owned or church-affiliated ones, may not be institutional members of the AHA, can they, their owners, or their administrators be morally compelled to abide by the AHA Code? Organizations such as the Federation of American Hospitals (FAH) and the Catholic Hospital Association (CHA) have ethical guide-

71

lines that differ somewhat from those of the AHA. Still others have either their own ethical codes or abide by other more general statements. For example, the Code of Ethics of the American College of Health Care Administrators (ACHCA) guides the behavior of administrators of long-term care facilities. In contrast, the American Health Care Association (AHCA) expects its members to abide by its generalized patients' bill of rights.

THE ETHICAL PRINCIPLE APPROACH

Another approach to categorizing ethical issues in health management focuses on fundamental ethical principles. Hiller (1984) has described five principles essential to resolving ethical dilemmas arising in health management --beneficence, nonmaleficence, respect for persons, justice, and utility. (See the preceding chapter "Ethical Decision Making and Health Administration" for a detailed discussion of these principles.)

Beneficence dictates that administrative actions ought to benefit those they affect. At a minimum, nonmaleficence states that such decisions ought to "do no harm." Respect for persons instructs decision makers to preserve the autonomy of individuals and to respect patients' right to self-determination. The principle of justice, which has many interpretations, demands administrative fairness and an equal distribution of risks and benefits. The principle of utility has a procedural meaning in that it calls for an orderly balance among the four other principles.

Since each of these principles can be applied at a macro, meso, or micro level, there are 15 possible permutations and combinations of principles and levels. Further complexity arises in that administrators may hold different priorities for different areas of accountability. Hence, attempts to classify ethical issues by relevant ethical principles would be limited at best.

THE COMBINED LAW AND ETHICS APPROACH

Henderson (1982) has developed another conceptual approach: quadrants of congruence and divergence in the relationship of law and ethics. By applying this model to issues in health management, Darr (1984) attempts to categorize problems as ethical, legal, or both.

Quadrant I consists of legal and ethical decisions and actions. Example actions include avoiding conflict of interest, refusing to use confidential information for personal gain, not embezzling, cooperating with other health care organizations, and encouraging comprehensive health services for the community.

In Quadrant II are issues that are viewed as ethical but illegal. For example, an administrator may take no action on learning that an increasing amount of morphine had been administered to relieve the pain of a terminally ill patient. Since this treatment also hastened the patient's death, it was technically illegal. However, as there was no intentional foul play involved, criminal charges most likely would not be pressed. Viewed from an ethical perspective, the act could be considered moral because it caused no real harm and may even have "done good" given the patient's prognosis and condition.

Quadrant III comprises activities that are legal but unethical. For instance, nonfederally funded surgical experimentation of questionable safety, the use of an informed consent form that fails to provide full disclosure of significant risks or omits alternative therapies, or failure to take administrative action against a surgeon who is only marginally qualified or who has an alcohol problem are all examples of legal but unethical actions.

Quadrant IV contains actions that are both unethical and illegal, such as bribing public officials, discriminating in hiring, or falsifying Medicare cost reports.

The major strength of the quadrant approach is that it forces a distinction between that which is legal/illegal and that which is ethical/unethical. However, it suffers from lack of universal interpretation and the ambiguous relationship between law and ethics. It presumes general agreement and understanding of the distinctions between that which is legal and that which is ethical, which is often not the case.

THE ENVIRONMENTAL FORCES ASSESSMENT APPROACH

Many ethical dilemmas in the health care industry have been attributed to various external forces; therefore, another approach to classification is to arrange these dilemmas according to major environmental influences responsible for the problem.

Prominent among those factors prompting ethical quandaries is government intervention through executive regulation, legislation, judicial opinions, and court orders. Community attitudes and values in our pluralistic society also create ethical problems that stem from social pressures and consumer expectations, demographic transitions (e.g., the aging of the population), and concerns about social equity and distributive justice.

Starr (1982, p. 514) has argued that the most significant force influencing the health care system is the emergence of multihospital corporations that have the size, political power, and profit motive to redirect the traditional mission of the industry. Pellegrino (1984, p. 40) has pointed to five major forces producing revolutionary changes--and ethical dilemmas--in the delivery of health care: (1) the technical revolution, (2) the pluralistic moral climate, (3) extensive media coverage, (4) political impact, and (5) economic factors. Hiller (1984, p. 160) has categorized four broad areas of external forces precipitating many of the ethical dilemmas confronting health administrators: (1) economics, government intervention, and public policy; (2) corporatization, the profit motive, and competition; (3) professionalism and increased professionalization; and (4) scientific and technological advances. Peters and Wacker (1982) have stressed the importance of conducting a sound environmental assessment for planning and marketing. They further emphasize that strategic planning and marketing must be rooted in values and ethics.

THE COMPETING INTEREST ACCOUNTABILITY APPROACH

Another approach to identifying ethical issues is based on the unique role filled by health administrators. According to Austin (1974, p. 316), health administrators frequently find themselves on the horns of a dilemma with regard to accountability because they must continually juggle a series of competing demands and responsibilities. He suggests a simple taxonomy of administrative accountability that includes six elements: (1) owner, (2) community, (3) consumer (patient), (4) resources, (5) regulatory, and (6) third party--any of which can conflict with personal values. While having to tackle these competing accountabilities, administrators remain morally bound to the codes of ethics of their profession and related associations.

An AHA Report: Values in Conflict

Recently, the AHA Special Committee on Biomedical Ethics discussed competing interests in hospital management, especially in the provision of patient care. In its final report, *Values in Conflict: Ethical Issues in Hospital Care* (1985), the Committee recognized the significance of clashing values in modern hospitals and advised hospitals to develop institutional policies and procedures relating to a range of ethical issues. In transmitting the report to the AHA General Council, Hofmann, Chair of the Committee, expressed the hope that the report would..."help hospitals to create an environment in which the ethical challenges in patient care delivery can be met in a compassionate and morally responsible manner that is sensitive to the needs of patients, their families, health care professionals, and the hospital (AHA, 1985, p.i).

75

In fulfilling this charge, administrators must balance competing needs as fairly as possible. The report (AHA, 1985, pp. 1-2) concluded,

> By virtue of its mission, its historical roots in charitable and religious organizations, and its fiduciary commitment to each patient and the community, the hospital is usually perceived to have a particular, if assumed, moral responsibility for health care. First, as a medical institution, the hospital has the responsibility for supervision and review of patient care. The hospital must ensure that standards of quality are met and make certain that the basic processes that characterize relationships and decisions between patients and health care professionals are consistent with sound ethical principles.
>
> Second, as a health care provider and an employer with a commitment to patient care, the hospital must develop policies and mechanisms through which questions of human values may be addressed. Third, as a center of health care delivery in the community, the hospital must respond responsibly to social problems and dilemmas that affect the demand and need for health care services.
>
> These roles all reinforce the need for a coherent, institution wide approach to ethical issues that arise in patient care.

The report acknowledges the need for sensitivity to the wide variety of values held by those who work for and are associated with the hospital, including its patients, their families, health professionals, patient representatives, chaplains, the community, members of the institution's governing body, administration, and medical staff.

While targeting mostly patient care issues, the report "is intended as a guide for hospital administrators, trustees, medical staffs, nurses, and other health care professionals." The Committee chose to focus on approaches to resolving conflicts rather than prescribing specific policies, although it recommends developing policies and practices related to several areas of ethical concern (see Table 5).

Balancing Competing Accountabilities

As described by Austin (1974), the AHA (1985), and others (Beauchamp and Bowie, 1983; Pellegrino and Thomasma, 1981), many ethical conflicts arise from the fact that administrators are accountable to multiple parties (interests) concurrently. While most administrators agree that their actions ought to be guided by the historical healing, or beneficent, mission of health care, they acknowledge often having to wrestle with competing obligations, which creates additional dilemmas. To the degree that they divert from this mission, administrators risk generating additional issues involving ethical dilemmas.

Balancing competing accountabilities can help identify and examine the sources of many ethical issues, although it is source-based (i.e., comprises specific issues) rather than theory- or principle-based. However, its strength lies in its relevance to, understanding of, and acceptance by administrators. It provides a taxonomy based on administrators' mutual and conflicting accountabilities.

The approach is comprehensive and organized, but it does have weaknesses. Some sources are closely associated with a particular level(s), yet most generate dilemmas in the meso level. Most troubling is that competing interests are not necessarily mutually exclusive; for example, some problems may "fit" into more than one source. Examples of dilemmas attributable to particular administrative accountabilities are given in Table 6.

Multiple interests create multiple conflicts. For example, adherence to sound management practice often challenges the traditional beneficent mission of the hospital. Sometimes community and consumer interests appear to be

77

TABLE 5   Recommended Areas for Hospital Policy and
           Practices Related to Biomedical Ethics
_____

Allocation of resources
Collaborative decision making
  Informed consent
  Barriers to capacity
  Assessment of capacity
  Role of minors
Confidentiality
Continuity of care
Do-not-resuscitate decisions
  Institutional review in cases of
    surrogate-physician disagreement
  Review of do-not-resuscitate decisions
Forgoing life-sustaining treatment
  Support for patient
  Support for families
Medical errors
Accommodations of moral convictions of employees
Provider competence
Restraints
Service mix selection
Technology acquisition

Policies Related to Biomedical Ethics Should:

  Be consistent with the institution's mission
  Be the basis for conflict resolutions regarding values
  Be sensitive to community standards
  Be the basis for educational programs
  Respect the patient's responsibility for decision
    making
  Support the appropriate roles of others in decision
    making
  Support an environment of information sharing and
    consultation on ethical questions
  Respect personal liberties
  Support conflict resolution at the level closest to
    the patient

_____

Source: Adapted, American Hospital Association (1985, p.
65).

TABLE 6   Competing Administrative Accountabilities

Owners

Owners establish an institution's mission and priorities. Administrators are held accountable for implementing the goals and objectives necessary to adhere to these priorities.

Community (Public)

A community in which an institution is located has expectations, based on shared values, about the services the institution should provide. Administrators are held publicly accountable for respecting community values and protecting the public's health and welfare.

Consumers (Patients and Families)

An institution's patients hold it accountable for maximizing the benefits accrued by the services provided. Since administrators are responsible for institutional policies, patients (and their families) often hold them personally accountable for what happens.

Profession

Administrators are individually accountable for upholding the standards of the profession as outlined in the Code of Ethics of the American College of Healthcare Executives. They are expected to reflect the values and behaviors that the profession expects of its members.

Medical Staff

Physicians are ethically bound to benefit their individual patients. Toward this end administrators are accountable for ensuring the availability of the necessary resources (such as medical technology) to facilitate the delivery of quality medical care by the medical staff.

Nursing Staff

Nurses, too, are bound by an ethical code. They are committed to caring for the sick, and administrators must respect their mission. Administrators are often called on to adjudicate conflicts between nurses and physicians.

Other Staff

Other professional and nonprofessional staff, who have a variety of interests and priorities, work in health institutions. Administrators are obligated to respect these staff members as individuals and deal with them fairly in all matters.

Third-Party Payers

Administrators are highly accountable to several third parties in fulfilling their responsibilities. For example, they must comply with the policies of a wide variety of third-party payers: Medicare, Medicaid, Blue Cross/Blue Shield, and commercial insurers. The paperwork can be daunting: substantiating claims for payment, audits for services and fees, monitoring quality and equality of care rendered, and assessing and controlling costs (Hiller and Seidel, 1982, p. 339).

Creditors

Administrators bear an ongoing obligation to ensure the financial integrity of their institutions. In doing so, they remain accountable to their creditors. They must keep their institutions in the black, keep the doors open, and maintain long-term solvency. They are thus responsible to the financial community for sustaining favorable credit ratings, interest rates, and access to capital.

Science and Technology

Research conducted in health care institutions has led to advances in medicine and biomedical technology. In therapeutic research (which may provide direct benefit to the patient/subject) the risk-benefit ratio is usually disclosed and justified. However, in nontherapeutic research, potential scientific advancements must be weighed against patient autonomy and safety. Administrators are often in a position to promote such research, but in so doing they face conflicts regarding their obligation to protect patients while encouraging research to advance the knowledge base of society. Hence, they bear a dual accountability to both researchers and subjects.

Education

Administrators are often teachers and mentors, such as when they serve as preceptors for interns or residents in health administration programs. In this capacity, they serve the profession, but they also face conflicts of accountability to academic programs, students, and their own institutions.

External Regulators (Rule Makers)

Administrators are accountable to external regulators, both governmental (e.g., Health Care Financing Administration, Occupational Safety and Health Administration, state rate-setting commissions, state licensure boards) and voluntary (e.g., Joint Commission on Accreditation of Hospitals, National Fire Protection Association). Compliance with various regulatory bodies often serves as a source of conflicting accountabilities.

Personal

Administrators bear a primary accountability to themselves. They must respect their own values, especially when these values conflict with those held by others. They need to believe in what they do.

sacrificed to owner or institutional priorities. And di-
emmas arise out of differences in institutional missions
as a result of owner differences and the prevalent "survival
of the fittest" atmosphere. In such institutions, "Administrators . . . should not restrict their role to attending
to bureaucratic concerns, but should insist on the moral
character of the institution" (Thomasma, 1982). Pellegrino
(1985) maintains that hospitals must not forget that their
first and foremost mission is to benefit patients, regardless of cost or profits.

The 51 Percent Minimum

The earliest hospitals, dating back to medieval times,
were places of healing and charity where the only purpose
was patient care (Rosen, 1963, pp. 2-3). Hospitals were
governed primarily, if not exclusively, by this humanistic,
charitable drive. In recent times, however, the roles
and responsibilities of health administration have grown
in number and in complexities, often forcing diversions
from the primary commitment to care. While ethical dilemmas
arise as a result of this, institutions must maintain no
less than a 51 percent commitment to their historical roots.
No other mission should be given higher priority than this
fundamental one. Should the charitable, healing mission
be overwhelmed by any other, such a position would be deemed
unethical.

AREAS OF ETHICAL CONFLICT IN HEALTH MANAGEMENT

To further facilitate analytical study and increased
understanding of ethical issues, it is helpful to categorize
major ethical dilemmas. However, such a classification
may not be comprehensive and does not preclude overlap:
specific ethical issues/problems can arise at more than
one of the three levels (micro, meso, and macro). Nevertheless, most dilemmas can be grouped primarily into one
of the 12 broad areas (or types) of concerns (see Table
7).

TABLE 7   A Basic Classification Scheme of
Ethical Issues in Health Management

Areas/Types of Concerns	Level of Ethical Issue		
	Micro	Meso	Macro
Institutional philosophy and mission			
Corporate ownership and tax status			
Community values and corporate (social) responsibility			
Ethics in management practice			
Economic and financial pressures			
Indigent care			
Research and technology			
Clinical and patient care issues			
Medical staff relations			
Staff relations			
Health administration as a profession			
Procedural issues			

Institutional Philosophy and Mission

This area focuses on problems associated with understanding institutional missions and priorities. It encompasses problems that arise in attempting to define the moral responsibilities of institutions and the degree to which they are viewed as pious platitudes or objectives developed to direct institutional operations.

Such conflicts frequently arise as administrators grapple with the degree to which health care institutions ought to remain bound to traditional healing and charitable missions in light of escalating challenges to institutional survival. Many of the issues classified in this area of concern arise in attempts to delineate authority between an institution's owners (or board of directors) and administrators. Some of the more common problems are associated with defining corporate philosophies and evolving strategic plans. For example, the degree to which an institution's mission statement emphasizes the traditional charity role of providing health care regardless of ability to pay, versus one that rations care due to profit seeking, often creates ethical conflict and precipitates heated debate. Some institutions espouse a religious mission, which implies a commitment to charity rather than profit (Pellegrino, 1985). Other elements of institutional missions often provoke different moral struggles. For instance, the refusal of Roman Catholic institutions to provide contraceptive information, abortion, or sterilizations contradicts the principle of respect for individual liberty that most nonsectarian institutions recognize.

Many academic medical centers are morally bound to a strong educational and/or research ideology. This revolves around a mission driven by a philosophical commitment to pursue new knowledge and to train future health care professionals, even at the expense of the healing mission.

Corporate Ownership and Tax Status

Ownership and tax status are closely related organizational entities. The law allows for both public and private institutions and for their operation as proprietary (for-profit) and voluntary (nonprofit) hospitals. Under existing law, nonprofit institutions get special tax considerations. Although such legal differences exist, the question remains of whether ownership and tax status should bear a certain moral character.

To some, the legal distinction of ownership is unclear, even exaggerated. Technically, it means that for-profit institutions may use some of their profit to pay dividends to their stockholders, whereas nonprofit institutions must channel all revenues back into their organizations. Despite this difference, "All hospitals must make a profit or close their doors. Nonprofit facilities call it unutilized resources or excess revenues, and the investor-owned companies call it profit" (Atkins, 1985, p. 69).

The fact that all institutions must make a profit to survive begs the central issue. Given the historical social mission of hospitals, the question really is whether they should be sufficiently "revenue rich" to make returns on investments beyond generating the necessary resources to keep them operating in good order. In other words, to what extent, if at all, is it morally permissible to profit from sick people?

Further questions frequently arise about whether different moral responsibilities should exist for public, private nonprofit, and private for-profit institutions? Does assumption of tax liability release for-profit institutions from other moral obligations? Do nonprofit institutions have additional moral obligations because they are tax-exempt? Should certain benefits be extended to institutions that accept all patients regardless of ability to pay?

People have widely divergent values about these issues. Some believe that for-profit health care is unethical.

Others say there is nothing wrong with it. The debate is complicated by multi-institutional arrangements in which both for-profit and nonprofit ventures exist under the same parent corporation. When discussing investor-owned health care corporations, O'Rourke (1984) claims that their goals and actions clearly do not correspond to the values traditionally embodied in the healing mission:

> Corporations in the field of medical care...
> must have the same primary goal as health care
> professionals: service to individuals in need
> of healing. . . . The corporation must maintain
> fiscal stability and make a profit, at the same
> time caring for those who cannot pay for help.
> . . . The ethical corporation does not use its
> profits to enrich investors, because this makes
> profit rather than service the good of the en-
> deavor. Moreover, taking money out of the medical
> care system makes it more expensive than it should
> be and often results in more affluent individuals
> profiting from the suffering of the less affluent.
> (pp. 18-19)

O'Rourke and others (Pellegrino, 1981, 1985; Relman, 1980, 1985; Young, 1984, 1985) suggest that ethical conflicts are generated by the very nature of the for-profit health care enterprise.

There are also strong arguments suggesting that the "focus on the 'investor-owned versus not-for-profit' question deflects attention from other issues that are more pertinent to the integrity of our health care system" (Williamson, 1984, pp. 27-28). Williamson says that the problems of the health care industry cut across ownership lines:

> The investor-owned hospital industry is an eco-
> nomic response to [the] new economic reality,
> rather than a "cause" of it. More and more
> not-for-profit hospitals are adopting the same
> corporate strategies and management methods used
> by investor-owned hospitals--i.e., they are em-
> ploying the same economic responses to the same

economic environment. As a result, the operating distinctions between investor-owned and not-for-profit hospitals are becoming so blurred that it is often difficult to tell them apart. (p. 28)

He further suggests that the real issue is the efficacy of the market system: "If a capitalistic health care model, as one part of our health care delivery system, can achieve social as well as financial objectives, i.e., do 'good' in addition to doing 'well,' this would be a far more productive inquiry than is the current controversy over ownership form as a predictor of behavior" (p. 28). He concludes,

Hospitals, regardless of ownership, are special kinds of institutions. They must meet both social and economic needs. In doing so, they must balance financial considerations with some less clearly defined social objectives. What is clear in this balancing act is [that] to meet social objectives, hospitals must first meet their financial needs. This applies to all hospitals regardless of ownership form. (p. 32)

With the erosion of the dominant structure of the community not-for-profit hospital and the growth of multi-institutional systems, the Institute of Medicine (1986) undertook a three-year study of the impact of such trends. Its report, *For-Profit Enterprise in Health Care*, marks the most comprehensive, authoritative assessment to date of the positive and negative implications of providing health care for profit. It concludes that "the debate about for-profit health care is fueled as much by values as by evidence" (Gray and McNerney, 1986, p. 1524).

Additional findings support the basis for much of the debate associated with differences in the priorities between for-profit and not-for-profit institutions. Based on somewhat inconclusive and often conflicting data that were available to the Institute of Medicine Committee,

such as the percentage of "uninsured patients" served and
the levels of "uncompensated care" provided, not-for-profit
hospitals appeared to provide more access to needed medical
care and a higher level of service than their for-profit
counterparts (Gray and McNerney, 1986, p. 1525). While
such differences might be explainable by factors other
than simply denying care to those unable to pay for it
(e.g., size or location of institution), "the majority
of the Committee agreed that the comparatively low levels
of compensated care in investor-owned hospitals that constitute 30 to 40 percent of the hospitals in a state suggest
that the presence of such hospitals lessens access to care
among people who lack means to pay" (Gray and McNerney,
1986, p. 1526).

The Committee acknowledged the social responsibility
of institutions, regardless of ownership, and upheld the
"traditional view of the basic moral purpose and mission
of health care institutions [that] begins with meeting
the needs of the sick" (Gray and McNerney, 1986, p. 1527).
Recognizing that the provision of needed medical care,
regardless of an ability to pay for it, has not always
been the first priority of all institutions, the report
"emphasizes the importance of putting the patient's interest
first," regardless of ownership status.

Other issues associated with institutional ownership
and affiliation are related to the locus of control and
authority of governing bodies. Private nonprofit, commu-
nity-based institutions are most often governed by elected
voluntary boards of directors, and some argue that they
are morally bound to reflect the values and priorities
of the community. In contrast, while governing bodies
of investor-owned institutions are also concerned with
community needs, they have an additional obligation to
make decisions that promote the best financial interests
of the corporation and its investors. While institutions
that are part of a large corporate network may have local
community input in their decisions, major decisions or
policy directives are often made in distant corporate board-
rooms. While ethical conflicts will arise regardless of
hospital ownership or locus of authority, the potential

for clashes between community and corporate interests increases as governing bodies are further removed from and less affected by the communities served by their institutions. Local community input is essential for institutions to reflect the dominant values in their environment.

Community Values and Corporate (Social) Responsibility

A rather wide array of ethical conflicts may be attributed to the perceived level of responsibility that corporations, including health care institutions, have for the communities they serve. At times, communities may hold unreasonable expectations about what institutions can (or should) do (or provide). For example, it is often asserted that institutions bear a special obligation to ensure unlimited health care as a right of all citizens. In other situations, issues arise in terms of the extent to which institutions are (or should be) bound to prevailing community norms that may reflect particular cultural, ethnic, or religious values.

Still other conflicts arise with respect to a corporation's social responsibility to its workers or to society in general. Classic examples involve safety in the workplace, product safety or quality, and air and water pollution. While laws often dictate minimum standards, worker or community expectations—or a sense of corporate responsibility—may demand more. Such issues are as relevant to health care institutions as to any other corporation, and possible even more so, given their common mission of promoting health and healing the sick.

If there is ample evidence that certain types of services are needed in a community, should an institution commit itself to making them available despite potential community resistance or objection? In turn, if sufficient need for certain types of care (e.g., skilled nursing, intermediate care facility beds, or psychiatric beds) cannot be demonstrated, should institutions be free to build such services knowing that in doing so community resources inevitably will be consumed? This question is at the heart of the debate between community planning and institutional (strategic) health planning advocates. It asks "Is certification of need (CON) morally valid?" (O'Sullivan and Hiller, 1981).

If an institution seeks the financial support of a community, does it bear certain moral obligations to that community? Does an institution that is the sole health care provider in a given area bear an added responsibility to meet the health care needs of the residents of that community?

As health care institutions increasingly operate as businesses, they must confront the difficult problems associated with the ethical dilemma of balancing profits and the broader social good. For example, should a hospital failing on economic grounds be closed? How do the governing bodies of such institutions and their administrators reckon with the catastrophic harm that such a move may bring a single-hospital town?

Davis (1975) contends that social responsibility arises from social power. In most communities, hospitals hold immense social power both as an employer and a provider of services. Such power dictates that the hospital administrators bear a social responsibility for their actions, which implies that in the process of managing health institutions, they are obliged to take actions that also protect and enhance society's interests. In addition, administrators bear responsibilities for social involvement in the areas of their competence where social needs exist. In other words, health administrators should contribute their knowledge and skills in helping to resolve community problems and engaging in community affairs. They ought not to remain isolated within their institutions. Friedman (1962) disagrees, arguing that in a free economy administrators possess only one social responsibility: serving the interest of their stockholders and maximizing their profits within the extent of the law. The moral dilemma for most administrators, however, is to determine a comfortable position along this continuum.

Within the business literature, cases abound that exhibit how corporations have wrestled with the issue of social responsibility. Some business executives exhibit a good deal of social consciousness. For example, according to McNerney (1985, p. 334),

> James Burke, chairman and chief executive officer of Johnson & Johnson, believes that a corporate credo "geared to service to society"--a credo in which people can believe--not only minimizes alien objectives, but leads to a better service or product; that is, it is better business. Johnson & Johnson's credo spells out responsibilities to customers, employees, communities, stockholders, in that order.

Johnson & Johnson demonstrated its high regard for corporate social responsibility during the Tylenol-cyanide episode in 1978, when it voluntarily acted to quickly remove Tylenol from the market until the package was redesigned to prevent tampering. The company bore a significant short-term financial loss in doing so. Seven years later there was another Tylenol-related death, and Johnson & Johnson again removed all Tylenol capsules from the market and announced that it would no longer offer the over-the-counter drug in capsule form.

In a similar action in 1980, Proctor and Gamble confronted the results of a Centers for Disease Control (CDC) study that revealed a strong correlation between the use of Rely tampons and toxic shock syndrome (which had killed 25 women since 1975). Although Proctor and Gamble never declared that its product was unsafe or defective, its own studies were unable to disprove the CDC findings. The company therefore withdrew a product that had been 20 years in development (Wokutch, 1983, p. 123). Proctor and Gamble's quick action was estimated to have cost it $75 million after taxes; however, its public reputation seems to have been largely redeemed.

Ethics in Management Practice

Within this category, many disparate issues involving ethics and values arise that confront health administrators and challenge generally agreed upon, ethically sound practices of institutional management. Some of the most serious and difficult ethical problems facing administrators result from conflicts of loyalty and conflicts of involvements, activities, and commitments outside their jobs that tend to bias their judgment on the job or motivate them to act in their own best interest (Graham, 1974, p. 90).

Although the range of possible ethics/values issues is broad, many involve adherence to the highly cherished ethical principles of justice and autonomy. Given the multiple parties to whom administrators are accountable, there is a clear need for them to be informed, fair, honest, rational, and responsible in their behavior and actions while always respecting others (namely, their employees, professional colleagues, and business associates).

Furthermore, the trust and credibility of health care institutions depends strongly on the professional competence and personal integrity of their administrators. Examples of activities in which ethical behavior often risks compromise in management practice include advertising and marketing, preparing and submitting reports, and communicating and negotiating with employees and business relations.

Where discretion exists, there is often uncertainty and possibly competing obligations and loyalties. In wrestling with such situations, administrators are "subject to a double hierarchy of authority, one impersonal and one personal, which define [their] obligations" (Graham, 1974, p. 90). Whereas the legal hierarchy is impersonal, the chain of command into which all administrators fall is quite personal. Administrators must interpret and delineate the law through policies, programs, instructions, rules, procedures, and a myriad of decisions. Neither the formal law nor the administrative law is always internally consistent (Graham, 1974, p. 91). As a result, many difficult ethical issues arise as attempts are made to resolve disagreements that grow out of different values, different degrees of ignorance or understanding, and different purposes. Thus, administrators must often meld various interpretations while using their own judgments and exercising their administrative authority. More specifically, it is important for administrators to inform others participating in decision making activities of any information pertinent to their role in the decision. Administrators should also carefully explain the rationale behind their final interpretations and decisions to avoid any misunderstandings or unnecessary distrust or conflict. They are bound to ensure that no personal conflict of interest has affected such decisions and to reveal any values that may have contributed to them.

Administrators must appreciate that value conflicts will arise in which they will have to defend decisions that they may personally reject, if these decisions have been made in accordance with the institution's mission, goals, and objectives. However, they should not engage in any unethical practices in achieving such ends, such as lying or being unjust. Should they ever confront a situation where they cannot accept a valid decision because it overwhelmingly compromises their personal values, the option of resignation should be considered.

Ethics once again bears on management practices in the responsibility of administrators to keep their promises, especially when contracts are involved (Bowie, 1982, p. 43), and in terms of administrative practices that would permit the marketing of unnecessary services or opportunities to make personal gains through conflicts of interest.

Coercion is an ever-present danger in hospital management, and while it is seldom discussed, enough concern has been expressed to make administrators sensitive to a wide range of actual and potential conflict inherent in their powerful positions. For example, is it ethical for administrators to benefit financially from their job-related decisions? Should administrators enter into contracts with firms of which they are an owner or investor?

Should they select patients, such as a kidney or liver recipient, because it might result in a large gift to the institution? To what lengths should an administrator go to prevent a conflict of interest between the institution and a member of the board, when doing so might jeopardize his own career? Must they always refrain from the not uncommon practice of awarding "sweetheart" contracts? For instance, if the hospital wants to sell a piece of its property, can it retain a real estate company owned by a member of the board? Again, administrators must be careful to distinguish between practices that are illegal and those that are unethical. While violating those which are illegal may carry the sanctions of law, those that are unethical should carry the force of professional and personal conscience.

Economic and Financial Pressures

Attempting to categorize the variety of economic and financial issues that precipitate ethical problems is difficult; some say that such pressures are the primary source of ethical dilemmas in health management and are so strong as to actually dominate moral considerations. Without question, an overwhelming prioritization of economic and financial factors diminishes or destroys the ability to recognize ethical problems or examine their implications. It simply strengthens what Ginzberg (1984) has referred to as the "monetarization of medical care."

Many of the major economic and financial issues have been grouped into four broad areas, none of which are mutually exclusive: (1) cost containment, (2) resource allocation, (3) competition and marketing, and (4) capital acquisition. Issues from each occur at all levels and affect a wide range of institutional and individual decisions. For example, eliminating one particular costly service may be a sound financial decision, yet it might provoke serious implications for the people who need the service.

Cost Containment

Efforts to contain costs are often unfair. While nearly everyone agrees that the skyrocketing costs of health care must be controlled, serious concerns arise over how this is to be achieved and to what extent such efforts will result in further inequities in the delivery of health care. To what degree does the adoption of a survival ethic or a profit drive result in ethical problems? Or, as Cunningham (1983) has asked, "Are hospitals forgetting their basic mission" in their struggle for institutional survival and marketplace gains? How, for instance, has the imposition of prospective reimbursement strategies, such as diagnosis-related groups (DRGs), created ethical dilemmas? Does it contribute to "patient dumping" or the premature discharge of patients still in need of care? Does elimination of cost shifting, a common practice under retrospective reimbursement, eliminate or curtail institutional care for the indigent? Clearly, such public policy shifts have raised both foreseeable and unforeseen ethical implications with which administrators must deal.

Mariner (1984, p. 243) has asked whether "DRGs provide appropriate criteria for a fair and efficient distribution of health care" Others (Dolenc and Dougherty, 1985; Stern and Epstein, 1985; Kapp, 1984; Omenn and Conrad, 1984) have raised serious questions about whether DRGs threaten to restrict access to health care, compromise quality, and impede development of medical technology. Recent hearings held by the U.S. Senate Special Committee on Aging (September-November 1985) have revealed significant negative implications of DRGs with respect to care of the elderly on Medicare.

If cost containment requires a balance between cost and quality, what is acceptable? To what extent can, or should, quality of care be justifiably sacrificed in saving money or generating revenue?

Resource Allocation

By acknowledging that resources are scarce and that choices must be made in allocating them, one inevitably faces ethical quandaries. And, in acknowledging that health care can be viewed as a commodity and that institutions compete to control market share, other significant issues emerge.

Decisions involving "macro" allocations (e.g., investments in advertising versus physical plant renovation versus support of money-losing services) generate questions. How should decisions be made about allocations for clinical services, such as breast cancer screening versus dental services versus organ transplantation? To what extent should such decisions attempt to benefit the greatest number? How should "micro" allocation decisions--for instance, who is to get the single artificial heart or the only available kidney--be made? Should these choices be made by administrators, physicians, or someone else? What rationale is used to decide what is most fair in allocation dilemmas?

Are administrators obligated to burden everyone equally with health care costs or only selected patients or groups? Is cost shifting justified because it shifts costs to those more able to bear the burden? Are cost-cutting strategies such as denying care to some individuals or eliminating costly services ethical? Is a multitiered health care system ethical, and if so, where should the lines be drawn and who should make such decisions? Kinzer (1984, p. 12) has suggested that "Acceptance of the idea of a two-tiered system of care seems to be gaining ground in our country, but only among those who know they will land safely in the top tier."

Competition and Marketing

Competition in health care, reinforced by government policies and withdrawal of government intervention, is increasing, creating serious ethical dilemmas (Gray, 1983,

p. 4). As health care increasingly becomes recognized as "big business," the rules of the marketplace encroach on its historical charitable healing mission, and institutions may sell or close unprofitable or overly costly facilities. As a result, communities are sometimes left to fend for themselves.

None should disagree that amid the growing competitive health care environment, innovative marketing strategies are crucial for institutional survival. Whereas hospitals used to operate in response to community needs (Rosner, 1982), they now respond to market pressures and sophisticated market analyses by using elaborate, creative, expensive advertising campaigns to lure new patients. Whether such practices are ethical is open to debate. Nonetheless, administrators are making decisions based on product choice, product line, and market share rather than real health needs, and ethical issues are arising.

Additional questions crop up as health care institutions use the high-powered marketing tools and tactics of other industries. Is it ethical to mislead or deceive consumers about their health care needs or the services provided by an institution? What ethical dilemmas arise as a result of one institution raiding the staff of another or establishing exclusive contracts with suppliers? What constitutes an appropriate mix of sensitivity to the community and legitimate institutional strategic planning? When is cooperation and joint planning with other health care institutions proper, and when is it not? Should antitrust concepts and laws apply in health care or should community and patient best interests prevail?

Capital Acquisition

Amassing capital also causes problems, and the degree to which an institution needs capital impinges on its financial decisions. For example, some institutions are forced to sacrifice needed services to improve their financial position to qualify for capital. This can be unjust to certain population groups.

Indigent Care

Serious ethical dilemmas arise with respect to ensuring justice and access to health care, and any discussion of these issues must include the needs of the poor. While the problems are accentuated by economic and financial concerns, the fundamental question is whether all people have a moral right, or claim to health care. Although the 1960s slogan that asks whether health care is a right or a privilege (for those who can afford it) is seldom seen today, and the Hill-Burton "free care" obligation is increasingly being fulfilled, the problem of indigent care remains and is receiving increased discussion.

To what extent, if any, might institutions abrogate the historical charitable mission of health care? Who should take responsibility for caring for the poor and uninsured? What ethical issues are generated by decreasing charity care through institution of policies such as mandatory preadmission screening, requirement of high deposits, and guarantee of prepayment or assurance of third-party coverage?

Assuming that a moral claim to health care exists (which is debatable by some), further problems arise in deciding who bears what responsibility for indigent care. Can institutions transfer patients for economic rather than clinical reasons? Should the government or the private sector be obligated to provide health care for the poor? If so, what are the limits of that obligation? What implications does the growth of for-profit health care have for the poor? Is it fair that public hospitals carry most of the burden of caring for the poor and uninsured?

Kinzer (1984, p. 5) has argued that other priorities have preempted concern for equity in health care delivery and forced moral and financial dilemmas on health care providers. If the burden falls on the poor themselves, they will simply not get the care they need. Many will suffer. Many will die. If institutions are forced to overly bear the burden, many will fold.

Situations such as those studied by the President's Commission on the Study of Ethical Problems in Medicine and Biomedical and Behavioral Research (1983) and reported by others (Iglehart, 1985; Mundinger, 1985; Wilensky, 1984; Knox, 1984; Wilensky and Berk, 1983) have documented denial of care to the poor and have generated serious concern throughout the industry and society. Everyone agrees that the problem is growing worse even as the debates rage on.

Research and Technology

The high cost of technological advances in medicine force hard choices on society, institutions, and individuals, most of which involve allocation problems regarding research and development. Most people agree that medical research is valuable and worthy of support, and most administrative decisions to authorize research reflect an intent to benefit individuals and society. In the case of major institutions, research also provides purpose, public recognition, visibility, and financial support. However, administrators must not lose site of the potential dangers and sacrifices of research. They are obligated to avoid preventable risk and discomfort to research subjects (who, when hospitalized or receiving therapy, are also patients), to assess the risk/benefit of proposed research, and to ensure that risks are fairly spread over the population and not centered on a particular group.

Administrators must also ensure the protection of subjects through support of and involvement in institutional review boards as prescribed under federal regulations. Moreover, they should understand the ethical principles underlying the conduct of research as developed by the U.S. Department of Health, Education, and Welfare's National Commission for the Protection of Human Subjects of Biomedical and Behavioral Research (1978) and summarized in the *Belmont Report*. The line between research and therapy is often unclear, but high standards must be imposed to ensure both the conduct of research and the protection of patient/subject welfare.

Motives for research can create problems, such as those recently dramatized by development of the artificial heart. Traditionally, research conducted at university-based medical centers permits pursuit of new knowledge wherever it may lead in the belief that researchers' only motive is discovery of the unknown to benefit humanity. Thus, academic institutions have enjoyed the benevolence of generous government grants. Individual recognition and prestige have always been seen as "frosting on the cake."

Public support for research is now dwindling, but some of the slack is being taken up by private investments. For example, Humana, Inc., launched a major artificial heart program, and although its executives have been commended for their tremendous commitment toward continuing the development of this technology in light of the government's withdrawal of support, they have also been criticized because of potential corporate financial gain and public recognition from the program. Critics claim that Humana's management of the media proves this, and others suggest that should the program not be profitable, Humana will drop it. We are also reminded that pharmaceutical companies and other biotechnology and bioengineering firms have a long history of pursuing research for purposes of financial and social gains. Nonetheless, the real question is whether it is ethical to make money from medical research, and on this point the debate continues.

Administrators must also face questions about the *type* of research they support. Genetic research, for example, can have far-reaching consequences for society.

Once technology has advanced from the research phase to be used therapeutically, other questions arise: Who will benefit from it (and live), and who will not (and die)? Institutions have only a limited amount of lifesaving equipment; how will it be allocated? And since all this technology is terribly expensive, how will hospitals absorb the cost of using it for patients who cannot afford it themselves? Are third-party payers obligated to pay for it?

Clinical and Patient Care Issues

Issues previously thought to concern only physicians are now seen as administrative problems as well. Hiller (1984, pp. 184-187) has observed that in the past, administrators avoided dealing with many such problems in attempts to not disrupt the physician-patient relationship. Indeed, some maintain that biomedical problems and patient care are not administrative matters. However, there are administrative aspects of many such issues. Administrators and their governing bodies must develop institutional policies and mechanisms through which ethical questions and value differences can be addressed.

As recommended by the American Hospital Association's Special Committee on Biomedical Ethics (1985) and shown in Table 1, there are several areas in which administration should become involved in solving physician-patient problems, such as forgoing life-sustaining treatment, ensuring informed consent and truth telling, and protecting confidentiality and privacy. For example, as medical information systems become more central to health care institutions, issues of disclosure and accessibility to patient records become more troublesome. Medical records are increasingly used for reasons other than provision of care, being sought for financial, research, quality assurance, legal, and other purposes. Administrators must establish and enforce policies designed to ensure patient's privacy, guarantee that patients are told the truth, and protect the integrity of the informed consent process by allowing the final treatment decisions (i.e., acceptance or rejection) to rest with the patients (assuming competency).

Medical Staff Relations

Hospitals and physicians have traditionally had a relationship that is both independent and interdependent. Overall, it has worked well but it has also caused problems. The origins of the professional values of the two entities differ: physicians are motivated by what is best for their patients and have little regard for cost, whereas administrators seek to achieve more utilitarian goals by acting in the best interest of the institution. Such an administrative orientation need not preclude benefiting individual patients, but it does favor that which the institution can provide to benefit the community at large.

Should administrators make decisions that favor the institution over individual patients? These conflicts clearly illustrate the common overlap of the micro, meso, and macro levels of ethical issues. Yet, all positions are founded on beneficent concerns, and therefore the tension maintains a dynamic balance. Nonetheless, this uneasy balance creates serious ethical issues for physicians (and other caregivers) and administrators, especially in view of the current shift in power toward administrators and their tighter control of purse strings. For example, to what extent should administrators assume control of matters that were heretofore in the medical domain? When do, or should, administrative concerns impinge on the provision of medical care, and will such intervention decrease the quality of care? And is there more or less conflict when physicians are also administrators?

As administrators try to gain increased cooperation among physicians in practicing more "cost conscious" medicine (e.g., increasing their efficiency), do they jeopardize the traditional physician-patient relationship? Should physicians be awarded financial bonuses for saving money for the hospital? Is it ethical to reward physicians for contributing to their institution's profitability? Should institutions and private physicians engage in profit sharing? According to Capron and Gray (1984),

> Increasing attention is being paid to arrangements by which hospitals would offer economic rewards to physicians whose patient care decisions help restrain the hospitals' expenses. Many hospitals are now developing plans by which physicians would share in the economic benefits when costs are kept under the DRG payment level. In addition to the "for-profit" hospitals that are playing an increasingly prominent role in American health

102

care, nonprofit hospitals are also exploring
how to develop incentive plans for physicians
without jeopardizing their tax-exempt status
. . . . We must ask, will it have undue negative
effects on patients and the health care system
as a whole?

Capron and Gray go on to warn that

Giving physicians a new financial interest in
the economic health of the hospital may weaken
the position of the physician as, first and foremost, the agent of the patient. Traditional
ethical norms dictate that a physician's primary
obligation is to patients, not to others--whether
they be relatives, institutions or even the physician's own welfare.

Is it ethical to induce physicians to admit certain
patients to one institution and other patients to another,
based on diagnosis, prognosis, expected length of stay,
or socioeconomic circumstance? What role should administrators have in determining whether certain physicians
practice in their institutions? Is it ethical for an institution to close its medical staff, or does that deny a
physician liberty and limit patient choice? Is it ethical
for institutions to make medical staff decisions based
on prevailing practice patterns and levels of individual
physician revenue generation for the hospital? How should
administrators deal with incompetent physicians? To what
extent should administrative concerns about costs and efficiency influence medical decision making? Are administrators responsible for the quality and competence of medical staff? Is the administrator or the institution bound
to support a physician should a case of alleged malpractice
arise? As the rise in medical malpractice insurance pre-
miums and judgments (i.e., court awards) are forcing some
physicians to limit their practices and/or to practice
defensive medicine, both of which are costly to patients
and society, should institutions assume the burden of providing such coverage?

These and other problems are causing increasing concern, and both administrators and physicians will have to reassess their respective roles and responsibilities. While it may be beneficial to move toward a more cooperative mission, neither group should lose sight of its own special ethical obligations. Administrators need to appreciate how hard it is for physicians to serve two masters. For as Levinsky (1984, p. 1575) has suggested, "It is to the advantage of our society and of the individuals it comprises that physicians retain their historic single-mindedness. The doctor's master must be the patient."

Staff Relations

Nonphysician members of the institutional work force maintain a more traditional employer-employee relationship. While some staff members have more professional autonomy than others, they tend to have little power over institutional affairs. Nonetheless, there are still ethical conflicts, mostly as a result of differences in personal values and perceived staff responsibilities. Sometimes the tension created by conflicts between individuals and the institution requires administrative intervention, which must be taken fairly and sensitively. For example, are health professionals and other nonprofessional staff always obligated to support the institution's mission? Institutional policies or medical practices can conflict with the personal values held by individual staff members and create morale and other personnel problems.

Other staff-related issues involve human resources and labor relations. Is it ethical for administrators to cut back staffing to an extent that quality of care may be lessened? What constitutes an appropriate response by clinicians (e.g., nursing staff) if cost-saving measures appear to impinge on patient care? Regardless of the legitimacy and the lack of other alternatives,) is it ethical for health care professionals to unionize, engage in collective bargaining, and/or strike? The latter activity generates serious ethical dilemmas since patients often become the pawns in labor disputes. When do the needs

of patients justify management intervention in staff conflicts or imposition of disciplinary action? Should staff
be allowed to refuse to jeopardize their physical welfare
especially when the danger is something they do not usually
encounter on the job? More specifically, may staff members
refuse to care for AIDS patients. What ethically justifiable action should administrators take in such cases?

Many of the ethical dilemmas involving staff relations
result from professional differences and interpretations.
Others seem to depend on the resolution of whether health
care professionals bear an added moral obligation to extend
themselves beyond what is expected in other industries
simply due to the fundamental healing mission of with their
profession.

Health Administration as a Profession

Beyond everything already discussed, some issues are
simply specific to or inherent in the profession of health
administration. While administrators are accountable to
more different interests (see Table 6) than they probably
find comfortable, the profession itself constitutes a par-
tial union of two paths that have traditionally borne dual
(and often competing) missions: business/management and
health care. As such, do health administrators have moral
obligations that their "pure" managerial counterparts in
other industries do not? And given the diverse backgrounds
and current positions of health administrators, are there
moral obligations common to the profession as a whole?
What is the source of such obligations, given the variety
of ethical codes possessed by the many different professional associations to which health administrators hold
allegiance? Are some conflicts created by lack of a single
professional association and single ethical code? Should
there be a substantive and enforceable code of ethics to
which all administrators are accountable? If so, what
would constitute a violation and how should violators be
punished? (For comparison, consider the medical profession's
wide acceptance of both the "Principles of Medical Ethics"

of the American Medical Association and the "Hippocratic Oath.")

By virtue of their individual and collective responsibilities, do health administrators bear an added level of social (or ethical) responsibility in attempting to guide the further development of the health care system and American health care policy? Given their knowledge and expertise, to what extent should administrators expend their time and energy in community and civic affairs? Should such commitments vary based on whether they are related or unrelated to the institution? Do administrators, particularly those from large teaching medical centers, have an obligation to commit their talents to promoting health care initiatives and policy development at the state and national levels, recognizing that such efforts will further remove them from their internal institutional responsibilities? Is it appropriate for administrators to assume active roles in political affairs, and if so, to what extent? Where is the line between expressing opinions that reflect the mission of one's institution and exercising one's individual beliefs in the political process? To what extent may these diverge before an individual's actions may be viewed as jeopardizing the institution? What should be the respective roles of the various professional associations and trade organizations in the public policy arena? Should they be strong advocates for certain health issues? Should they collectively represent the interests of their respective members? Should they represent the public interest?

Procedural Issues

Procedural issues arise most often after the existence of an ethical dilemma has been acknowledged. They tend to be concerned with the question: "Who should decide?" Many procedural issues can be solved by established institutional policies, criteria, or standards. For instance, when may organs be removed for transplantation? When are no further resuscitation or artificial life support efforts

106

in order? Or, when are patient transfers justified or required?

When there is no policy, however, things get complicated, and alternative structures are often imposed. For example, unresolvable dilemmas frequently wind up in the courts amid complex, emotional, adversarial proceedings. While such an approach may be successful in producing a legal response to a problem and limiting potential liability, it does not necessarily resolve the ethical and moral dilemmas at hand. In matters involving the use of human subjects in biomedical and behavioral research, institutions employ institutional review boards (IRBs). Mandated by federal regulations, IRBs serve as a means to ensure adequate protection for subjects being used in human experimentation. They assess the inherent risks and potential benefits of proposed research and ensure that adequate informed consent procedures will be used and that the selection of subjects (patients) will be done in a fair manner.

While IRBs were designed to deal with ethical issues associated with research, institutional ethics committees (IECs) were established to assist in resolving a variety of ethical dilemmas encountered in patient care. As initially conceived, IECs had limited scope and were often referred to as "prognosis committees," whose purpose was to deal largely with questions concerning the terminally ill (i.e., whether life support should be discontinued). Such a role also earned them the title of "god squads," since they were called on to decide when a patient would die or which patient might live by being selected to receive a transplant. They achieved particular significance after the decision in the Karen Ann Quinlan case, when the court said a final decision should have the concurrence of an ethics committee. Increasingly, IECs have become viewed in a much broader context in terms of their activities and responsibilities.

More and more hospitals have been turning to IECs typically comprising a diverse membership of physicians, nurses, social workers, philosophers (medical ethicists), and clergy, among others. After a period of training,

IECs may assume both advisory and consultative roles for administrators, clinical staff, and patients and their families. Using various models of ethical decision making, IECs examine a problem, exploring all options (alternatives), implications for the multiple parties affected, and conflicting values, and then attempt to generate recommendations that are ethically justifiable based on the unique situations at hand.

As a product of the 1984 Amendments to the Child Abuse and Neglect Prevention and Treatment Act (P.L. 98-457) and its associated regulations published in April 1985, guidelines for treating and reporting severely disabled newborns were established. While such guidelines had previously existed in some institutions, these regulations gave considerable attention to a special type of IEC known as an infant care review committee (ICRC), charged with specifically reviewing cases in which the withdrawal of life-sustaining treatment of severely defective newborns might be considered.

Mounting experience suggests that IECs and ICRCs are playing increasingly significant roles in resolving ethical issues involving patient care. Another approach used primarily by large teaching hospitals is to hire ethicists (typically doctorally prepared philosophers who may be members of the teaching faculties at universities or medical schools). Such individuals provide ongoing consultation with clinical staff on a wide array of ethical issues. Both IECs and staff ethicists can provide assistance to administrators in their deliberations over ethical problems of an administrative nature. They may be particularly helpful in making resource-allocation decisions, resolving conflicts of interest, and deriving institutional policies related to patient care (e.g., informed consent, information disclosure to third parties).

However, in the absence of ethics committees or staff ethicists to help them wrestle with ethical issues, administrators must be prepared to exercise their own decision making skills, to secure the needed assistance of others to help them work through the actual decision making process, or to delegate this responsibility to those equipped to do so.

SUMMARY

As resources grow increasingly scarce and competition, efficiency, and technology advance as the dominant driving forces in the health care system, the plethora of ethical issues confronting today's health administrators become ever more varied and complex. The issues facing administrators range from such dramatic ones as forgoing life support and denying medical care to persons unable to pay for it to ones that are more characteristic of the "nitty-gritty, day-to-day snap judgment kind of decisions" that all administrators make but that also have important ethical implications (May, 1975). It is this latter type of decision which, when made individually, seems almost insignificant, but that when viewed collectively reflects an ethical posture that shapes and molds health care institutions and the services they deliver.

This chapter has illustrated some of the complexities with which health administrators must struggle, many being magnified due to their concomitant accountability to multiple interests. It identified both substantive issues for which facts and values are often intermingled, and procedural questions, which are often raised in terms of who should decide. More specifically, it has provided an array of various old and new frameworks from which ethical issues may be examined. In addition, a topical issue/problem-oriented system for classifying ethical dilemmas has been created and discussed in the context of an imperfect matrix consisting of three overlapping and often competing levels (i.e., macro, meso, and micro).

Administrators are encouraged to remain sensitive to five fundamental normative ethical principles as they approach the wide array of moral dilemmas associated with their work. However, no effort has been or should be made to dictate the results of their deliberations. Rather, the ability to identify the myriad ethical issues they will confront in their work and the tools they need to tackle them should equip administrators to meet the challenges of health administration today and tomorrow.

References

American College of Hospital Administrators. *Code of Ethics*. Chicago, Ill.: American College of Hospital Administrators, 1980.

American Hospital Association. *Values in Conflict: Ethical Issues in Hospital Care, Report of the Special Committee on Biomedical Ethics*. Chicago, Ill.: American Hospital Association, 1985.

American Hospital Association and American College of Hospital Administrators. *Code of Ethics*. Chicago, Ill.: American Hospital Association, 1941, 1957.

Atkins, George. As quoted in Jack Bleich, "Profit, non-profit hospitals differ in views on values, competition." *Medical Ethics Advisor* 1(5):69-70, June 1985.

Austin, Charles J. "What is health administration?" *Hospital Administration* 19:14-29, Summer 1974.

Beauchamp, Tom L., and Norman E. Bowie. *Ethical Theory and Business*, 2nd edition. Englewood Cliffs, N.J.: Prentice-Hall, 1983.

Beauchamp, Tom L., and Laurence B. McCullough. *Medical Ethics: The Moral Responsibilities of Physicians*. Englewood Cliffs, N.J.: Prentice-Hall, 1984.

Bowie, Norman. *Business Ethics*. Englewood Cliffs, N.J.: Prentice-Hall, 1982.

Capron, Alexander M., and Bradford H. Gray. "Between you and your doctor." *Wall Street Journal*, February 6, 1984.

Cunningham, Robert M., Jr. "More than a business: are hospitals forgetting their basic mission?" *Hospitals* 57:88-90, January 16, 1983.

Darr, Kurt. "Administrative ethics and the health services manager." *Hospital and Health Services Administration* 29(2):120-136, March/April 1984.

Davis, Keith. "An expanded view of the social responsibility of business." *Business Horizons* 28(3), June 1975.

Dolenc, Danielle A., and Charles J. Dougherty. "DRGs: the counterrevolution in financing health care." *Hastings Center Report* 15(3):19-29, June 1985.

Friedman, Milton. "The social responsibility of freedom." In Milton Friedman, *Capitalism and Freedom*. Chicago, Ill.: University of Chicago Press, 1962, pp. 133-136.

Ginzberg, Eli. "The monetarization of medical care." *New England Journal of Medicine* 310(18):1162-1165, May 3, 1984.

Graham, George A. "Ethical guidelines for public administrators: observations on rules of the game." *Public Administration Review* 34(1):90-92, January/February 1974.

Gray, Bradford H. "An introduction to the new health care for profit." In Bradford H. Gray, ed., *The New Health Care for Profit: Doctors and Hospitals in a Competitive Environment*. Washington, D.C.: National Academy Press, 1983, pp. 1-16.

Gray, Bradford H., and Walter J. McNerney. "For-profit enterprise in health care: the Institute of Medicine Study," *New England Journal of Medicine* 314(23):1523-1528, June 5, 1986.

Greenwood, E. "Attributes of a profession." *Social Work* 2(3):44-55, July 1957.

Henderson, Verne E. "The ethical side of enterprise." *Sloan Management Review*, Spring 1982, pp. 37-47.

Hiller, Marc D. "Medical ethics and public policy." In Marc D. Hiller, ed., *Medical Ethics and the Law: Implications for Public Policy.* Cambridge, Mass.: Ballinger Publishing Company, 1981, pp. 3-45.

Hiller, Marc D. "Ethics and health care administration: issues in education and practice." *Journal of Health Administration Education* 2(2):147-192, Spring 1984.

Hiller, Marc D., and Lee F. Seidel. "Patient care management systems, medical records, and privacy: a balancing act." *Public Health Reports* 97(4):332-345, July/August 1982.

Iglehart, John K. "Medical care of the poor: a growing problem." *New England Journal of Medicine* 313(1):59-63, July 4, 1985.

Institute of Medicine. *For-Profit Enterprise in Health Care.* Washington, D.C.: National Academy Press, 1986.

Kapp, Marshall B. "Legal and ethical implications of health care reimbursement by Diagnosis Related Groups." *Law, Medicine, and Health Care* 12(6):245-253, 278, December 1984.

Kinzer, David M. "Care of the poor revisited." *Inquiry* 21:5-16, Spring 1984.

Levey, Samuel, and James Hill. "Between survival and social responsibility: in search of an ethical balance." *Journal of Health Administration Education* 4(2):225-231, Spring 1986.

Levinsky, Norman G. "The doctor's master." *New England Journal of Medicine* 311(24):1573-1575, December 13, 1984.

Mariner, Wendy K. "Diagnosis related groups: evading social responsibility?" *Law, Medicine, and Health Care* 12 (6):243-244, December 1984.

May, J. Joel. "Introductory remarks." In *Ethical Issues in Health Care Management: Proceedings of the Seventeenth Annual Symposium on Hospital Affairs*. Chicago, Ill.: University of Chicago, Graduate Program in Hospital Administration and Center for Health Administration Studies, Graduate School of Business, April 1975, pp. 1-2.

McNerney, Walter J. "Managing ethical dilemmas." *Journal of Health Administration Education* 3(3):331-340, Summer 1985.

Mundinger, Mary O. "Health service funding cuts and the declining health of the poor." *New England Journal of Medicine* 313(1):44-47, July 4, 1985.

Neuhauser, Duncan. *Coming of Age: A 50-Year History of the American College of Hospital Administrators and the Profession It Serves, 1933-1983*. Chicago, Ill.: Pluribus Press, 1983.

Omenn, Gilbert S., and Douglas A. Conrad. "Implications of DRGs for clinicians." *New England Journal of Medicine* 311(20):1314-1317, November 15, 1984.

O'Rourke, Kevin. "An ethical perspective on investor-owned medical care corporations." *Frontiers of Health Services Management* 1(1):10-26, September 1984.

O'Sullivan, Michael J., and Marc D. Hiller. "Ethics and health planning." In Marc D. Hiller, ed., *Medical Ethics and the Law: Implications for Public Policy*. Cambridge, Mass.: Ballinger Publishing Company, 1981, pp. 73-92.

Pellegrino, Edmund D. "Ethical issues in a competitive environment." *Hospital Forum*, July/August 1984, pp. 40-41.

Pellegrino, Edmund D. "Catholic hospitals: survival without moral compromise." *Health Progress* May 1985, pp. 42-49.

Pellegrino, Edmund D., and David C. Thomasma. *A Philosophical Basis of Medical Practice: Toward a Philosophy and Ethic of the Health Professions*. New York: Oxford University Press, 1981, pp. 244-265.

Peters, Joseph P., and Ronald C. Wacker. "Strategic planning must be rooted in values and ethics." *Hospitals* 56(11):90-98, June 16, 1982.

President's Commission on the Study of Ethical Problems in Medicine and Biomedical and Behavioral Research. *Securing Access to Health Care: The Ethical Implications of Differences in Availability of Health Services*. Washington, D.C.: U.S. Government Printing Office, 1983.

Reinhardt, Uwe E. "Hard choices in health care: a matter of ethics." In Lynn Etheredge, Uwe E. Reinhardt, Theodore R. Marmor, Andrew Dunham, Karen Davis, and David Blumenthal, *Health Care: How to Improve It and Pay For It*. Washington, D.C.: Center for National Policy, April 1985.

Relman, Arnold S. "The new medical industrial complex." *New England Journal of Medicine* 303(17):963-970, October 23, 1980.

Relman, Arnold S. "Cost control, doctors' ethics, and patient care." *Issues in Science and Technology* I:103-111, Winter 1985.

Rosen, George. "The hospital: historical sociology of a community institution." In Eliot Freidson, ed., *The Hospital in Modern Society*. New York: Free Press of Glencoe, 1963, pp. 1-36.

Rosner, David. *A Once Charitable Enterprise: Hospitals and Health Care in Brooklyn and New York, 1885-1915.* New York: Cambridge University Press, 1982.

Starr, Paul. *The Social Transformation of American Medicine.* New York: Basic Books, Inc., 1982.

Thomasma, David C. "Hospitals' ethical responsibilities as technology, regulation grow." *Hospital Progress* 63:74-79, December 1982.

U.S. Department of Health, Education, and Welfare, The National Commission for the Protection of Human Subjects of Biomedical and Behavioral Research. *The Belmont Report: Ethical Principles and Guidelines for the Protection of Human Subjects of Research.* Washington, D.C.: U.S. Government Printing Office, September 30, 1978. DHEW Publication No. (OS) 78-0012.

U.S. Senate Special Committee on Aging. *Impact of Medicare's Prospective Payment System on the Quality of Care Received by Medicare Beneficiaries: Staff Report.* September 26, 1985.

U.S. Senate Special Committee on Aging. *Impact of Medicare's Prospective Payment System on the Quality of Care Received by Medicare Beneficiaries: Staff Report.* October 24, 1985.

U.S. Senate Special Committee on Aging. *Medicare DRGs --The Government's Role in Ensuring Quality: Staff Report.* November 12, 1985.

Veatch, Robert M. "Ethical dilemmas of for-profit enterprise in health care." In Bradford H. Gray, ed., *The New Health Care for Profit: Doctors and Hospitals in a Competitive Environment.* Washington, D.C.: National Academy Press, 1983, pp. 125-152.

Wilensky, Gail R. "Solving uncompensated hospital care." *Health Affairs* 3(4):50-62, 1984.

Wilensky, Gail R., and M. L. Berk. "Poor, sick, and uninsured." *Health Affairs* 2(2):91-95, 1983.

Williams, David G. Jr. "Investor-owned versus not-for-profit hospitals: what are the issues?" *Frontiers of Health Services Management* 1(1):27-32, September 1984.

Wokutch, Richard. "Proctor and Gamble and toxic shock syndrome." In Tom L. Beauchamp and Norman E. Bowie, *Ethical Theory and Business*, 2nd edition. Englewood Cliffs, N.J.: Prentice-Hall, 1983, pp. 123-124.

Wrenn, Keith. "No insurance, no admission." *New England Journal of Medicine* 312(6):373-374, February 7, 1985.

Young, Quentin D. "Impact of for-profit enterprise on health care." *Journal of Public Health Policy* 5(4): 449-452, 1984.

Young, Quentin D. "The danger of making serious problems worse." *Business and Health* 2(3):32-33, January/February 1985.

APPENDIX A

Guidelines on Ethical Conduct and Relationships for Health Care Institutions

Adopted by the American Hospital Association and the American College of Healthcare Executives

Health care institutions are service organizations that provide patient care and a varying range of education, research, public health, and social services for their communities. These institutions carry public responsibilities for their own conduct, the health care of their patients, and the health of their communities. This role places special obligations upon health care institutions and their representatives to adhere to ethical principles of conduct. The following guidelines are intended to assist members of the American Hospital Association in defining their institutional policies, ethical relationships, and practices.

1. Health care institutions should be interested in the overall health status of people in addition to providing direct patient care services.

2. The public has accorded high priority to the availability of services to the sick and injured, but there are limits to the individual and collective resources available for this purpose. Recognizing this, health care institutions should support the most effective use of economic and other resources to ensure access to comprehensive health care services of high quality.

3. The community's health objectives are advanced when all health care providers and social, welfare, educational, and other agencies work together in planning and offering improved services. Health care institutions should promote and support such cooperation [ref 1].

4. Patient care services are inherently personal in nature. Health care institutions should maintain organ-

izational relationships, policies, and systems that are conducive to humane and individualized care for those being served.

5. Health care institutions, wherever possible and consistent with ethical commitments of the institution, should ensure respect and consideration for reasonable accommodation of the individual religious and social beliefs and customs of patients, employees, physicians, and others.

6. Health care institutions should establish and maintain internal policies, practices, standards of performance, and systematic methods of evaluation that emphasize high quality, safety, and effectiveness of care.

7. Health care institutions, being dependent upon community confidence and support, should accept an ethical sense of public accountability; reflect fairness, honesty, and impartiality in all activities and relationships; manage their resources prudently; and ensure that reports to the public are factual and clear in interpreting institutional goals, status, and accomplishments.

8. Health care institutions should relate to their communities and to each other constructively and in ways that merit and preserve public confidence in them, both individually and collectively.

9. Health care institutions that operate on a non-profit basis should feel free to publicize their various tax-exempt purposes that are deserving of charitable and philanthropic support [ref 2]. This may include an ongoing program of public relations and may range from reminders of the opportunities for memorials and charitable bequests to the conduct of a fund drive for a particular purpose. In responding to charitable and philanthropic interests or in soliciting contributions, health care institutions should not capitalize on the sensitivities of individuals in any way that might subject the institution's motivations to ethical criticism. Likewise, in directing such publicity to those who may be in the chain of providing goods and services to the institution, care should be taken to ensure

that the institution's approach complies with any legal restrictions on this activity [ref 3], does not suggest a relation to patronage that would support adverse reimbursement consequences, and precludes any suggestion that future patronage by the institution would be affected by charitable or philanthropic generosity. The demonstration of ethical commitment by the health care institution may well be the strongest assurance of continued charitable and philanthropic support.

References

1.   See *Statement on Health Planning*, AHA no. S025, 1976.
2.   See *Guidelines on Advertising by Hospitals*, AHA no. G030, 1977.
3.   Review should be made of possible technical violations of the Medicare-Medicaid Anti-Fraud and Abuse Act (P.L. 95-142) and similar legislation. Also see *Guidelines on Resolution of Conflicts of Interest in Health Care Institutions*. AHA no. G004, 1975.

APPENDIX B

Code of Ethics

Developed by a special Committee on Ethics,
Endorsed by the Board of Governors, and
Approved by the Council of Regents at its
Annual Meeting in Chicago on August 20, 1973.

American College of Healthcare Executives

PREFACE

The Code of Ethics is administered by the Committee
on Ethics, which is appointed by the Board of Governors
upon nomination by the Chairman. It is composed of nine
Fellows of the College, each of whom serves a three-year
term on a staggered basis, with three members retiring
each year.

The Committee on Ethics shall:

o   Review and evaluate annually the Code
     of Ethics, and make any necessary recom-
     mendations for updating the Code.

o   Review and recommend action to the
     Board of Governors on allegations
     brought forth regarding breaches of
     the Code of Ethics.

o   Refine the Code of Ethics to specific
     applications and to relate the Code
     to several membership classifications
     as compared to the Code for hospitals
     as institutions.

o   Prepare a report of observations, accom-
     plishments, and recommendations to
     the Board of Governors at the annual

reporting session, and such other peri-
odic reports as required.

The Committee on Ethics invokes the Code of Ethics
under authority of the ACHE *Bylaws*, Article II, Membership,
Section 8, b, Termination of Membership, as follows:

Membership may be terminated by action of the Board
of Governors as a result of violation of the Code of Ethics,
nonconformity with the Bylaws or Regulations Governing
Admissions and Advancements or conduct unbecoming a member.
No such termination of membership shall be effected without
affording a reasonable opportunity for the member to consider the charges and to appear in his defense before the
Board of Governors or its designate hearing committee.
The procedures for initiation, notification, and conduct
of such hearing shall be adopted by the Board of Governors.

PREAMBLE

An expected condition of affiliation with the American
College of Healthcare Executives is that the individual's
behavior will be ethical as a way of life in the conduct
of personal and business affairs.

Inherent in any human dealings are the possibilities
of unethical behavior in a variety of forms. The environment of health institutions and related programs presents
complex and unique settings of human relationships, replete
with potentials for behavior in conflict with desired ethical standards and projects consequences contrary to a
favorable public image.

The preceding demands that all ACHE members, and others, who bear any responsibility in the administration
of hospitals, other health institutions and related programs, remain constantly on the alert for the potentials
of unethical behavior that exist. Furthermore, that they
are prepared to undertake a sound and sober approach to
the solution of problems threatening to demean the public's
respect and acceptance of them as professionals in the

121

management of programs for the provision of health as well as of the enterprise with which they are associated.

The ACHE Code of Ethics is specifically designed to define and set forth broad guidelines applicable to the personal (professional) accountability of all members of the top-level management involved in the administration of hospitals, other health institutions, and related health activities represented in the mix of its membership. It is united in purpose with the Code of Ethics of the American Hospital Association, which defines standards of conduct for health institutions.

The purpose of the ACHE Code of Ethics is to attempt to assure and facilitate accomplishment of the goals of health institutions and programs through the integrity, skills, and impartiality of practitioners in the field of health administration.

Effective executive functioning and leadership demands the highest standards of ethical performance. This must occur not only within the corporate organizational structure itself but in the essential relationships with a multiplicity of institutions and agencies involved nowadays in the direct provision of health services or supportive thereto. Consequently, a duality of interests exist for the individual: one, personal, and the other as a representative of an organization serving as a major component of the overall health services system required to fulfill the needs of all the people.

The duality of interest identified confronts even the most conscientious ACHE member from time to time, with issues which pose difficult decisions and no clear cut courses of action. This applies similarly to members of the College occupying positions in the organization's top-management hierarchy other than those of chief executive officer. They face ethical issues and potential problems of a related but perhaps differing nature. The College's Code of Ethics is intended to apply equally to _all_ of the membership, regardless of their positions in administrative practice.

122

I. ACCOUNTABILITY

Health services administrators must meet two primary accountabilities--one as a member of the College, and the other in activities performed as an institutional executive.

A. It is expected that the *Guidelines on Ethical Conduct and Relationships for Health Care Institutions* (see Appendix II) as formulated by the American Hospital Association will be adhered to for the executive's institutional accountability:

1. Recognize that the care of the ill and injured is a prime responsibility and at all times strive to provide to all in need of health services quality care and treatment consistent with available resources.

2. Maintain and promote interpersonal relationships within the organization that will assure a supportive environment conducive to humane and appropriate care for those served.

3. Seek to merit the confidence and respect of patients and community through the quality and scope of services.

4. Extend consideration and respect for the social and religious practices and customs of patients, employees, and others to the maximum extent possible.

5. Stimulate, innovate, and encourage comprehensive health services.

6. Cooperate with other entities, engaged in or supportive of health services, to promote accessibility and the conduct of quality health programs.

7. Initiate support endeavors designed to ease the financial burdens of health care on an equitable basis for all patients and other individuals who need help in the solution of health problems.

8. Reports to the public should include factual information and interpret clearly institutional status, accomplishments, and objectives.

9. Fairness, honesty, and impartiality in all professional activities and relationships should be a prime focus of emphasis.

10. Maintain management and professional policies, practices, standards of performance, as well as activities for surveillance by measures for assessment, to assure quality in services provided and safe functional facilities.

B. In matters of professional and personal ethics, the administrator has a duty to:

1. Exercise the best in administrative judgment and skill for the benefit of the health services organization.

2. Maintain a standard of personal conduct solely directed toward promoting the best interests of the hospital, other health facilities or programs.

3. Observe at all times the existing local, state, and federal laws as a minimum guide for the fulfillment of responsibilities assigned.

4. Satisfy the duty of loyalty and fidelity in pursuit of the best interests of the hospital.

5. Conduct dealings on behalf of, and within the hospital in a manner that is honest and ethical, exercise administrative behavior in good faith to maintain confidence in administrative decisions.

6. Not use knowledge gained in performance of his duties nor make use of inside information for personal benefit which may be detrimental to the institution or the community served.

7. Not accept favors that will influence any decisions.

8. Not invoke any part of this Code of Ethics for selfish reasons.

II. THE GOVERNING BODY

Effectiveness in administrative performance depends upon mutual respect and harmonious relationships between the hospital administration and the governing authority. Such accord can be maintained best when the functions and prerogatives of each are carefully defined, understood, and followed.

A. The hospital executive in the fulfillment of defined functions and obligations shall:

1. Exercise the necessary authority assigned for conducting the affairs of the organization in all of its various activities and operating units in accordance with the policies adopted by the governing authority.

2. Manifest personal integrity and a high level of professional standards with capable leadership deserving of confidence and respect.

3. Consider as a major factor the interest of the organization and its community relations in all matters affecting the conditions of his employment.

III. THE MEDICAL STAFF

In organizations having a medical staff, hospital administration shall foster effective channels for the exchange of thinking and decision making among the governing board, the medical staff and administration.

A. To effect the above, the operating executive officer shall:

1. Provide coordination, support, and understanding in assisting the medical staff to accomplish its responsibilities and activities.

2. Enforce through appropriate channels the policies established for the welfare of patients and the continued effectiveness of the organization.

3. Evidence considerate and helpful assistance to members of the medical profession in the community who are not members of the medical staff, and encourage them to participate in hospital activities for continuing education within guidelines determined by the medical staff.

IV. AGENCY RELATIONSHIPS

Health service administration shall maintain a spirit of cooperation with representatives of other health care organizations where there is a sharing of common objectives.

A.   Fulfillment of this responsibility requires:

1. Assistance to other administrators and their organizations through participation in activities and services which will improve the quality of health care services and programs, and enhance the effectiveness and economy of the health care system.

2. Cooperation with education and planning organizations that contribute to the advancement of health care.

V. CONFLICT OF INTEREST

Health services administrators shall conduct their personal and professional relationships in such a way as to assure themselves, their organizations, and communities that decisions made are for the best interest of the organization without the slightest implication of wrong doing. The exercise of judgment is required to determine if a potential conflict of interest situation exists. A conflict of interest exists when an administrator is in a position, apart from the remuneration which he receives from his employment, to profit directly or indirectly through the application of his administrative authority or knowledge. Also, a conflict of interest exists if a friend or relative benefits, or the organization is adversely affected in any way by the administrative action.

Conflict of interest may be only a matter of degree between acceptable and unacceptable behavior.

A. Obligations

The administrator shall endeavor to avoid conflict of interest by:

1. Providing full disclosure to the governing authority of any potential conflict of interest before consummation of the transaction.

2. Making available annually to his governing authority a statement of his holdings, interests, or investments which might possibly be interpreted as a conflict of interest in the administration of a health services organization.

3. Avoiding any transaction where a conflict of interest is apparent.

4. Promptly informing the governing authority of any knowledge of potential conflicts of interest by other persons in the organization.

5. Permitting no commercial exploitation of his position.

6. Eliminating any possibilities of personal conflict of interest by:

   a. Divestiture of outside interest which can be suspected of being contrary to the expected conduct of his position responsibilities.

   b. Full and frank disclosure of any potential conflict of interest.

c. Resignation of his administra-
    tive position when the only
    acceptable alternatives war-
    rant such action.

d. Seeking guidance from his
    governing authority when
    any question arises about
    conflict of interest.

e. Obtaining direction from
    the ACHE Committee on Ethics
    regarding the application
    of the Code of Ethics as
    a guide for personal con-
    duct.

7. Removing any direct or indirect influ-
    ence on decision making that is in
    violation of this Code of Ethics.

B. Business Dealings

In business transactions for the hospital, an administrator shall not accept anything of substantial value from
a third party. Any benefit offered in the expectation
of influencing an administrator's judgment falls into this
class.

C. Systems Conflicts

Because of the need to coordinate and plan the operation of the larger health care system, administrators often
are elected and appointed to the governing authorities
of health-related organizations, such as planning bodies,
Blue Cross boards, state and national hospital associations,
and other health care organizations.

Inherent in such positions is potential conflict of
interest because of the duality of interests of the administrator. Such duality of interest is acceptable where there
is no conflict of interest. When duality of interest poses

a potential conflict of interest, full and frank disclosures must be made promptly. Participation in decision making, where a conflict of interest exists or can reasonably be construed, acceptable behavior requires that there be no further participation in decision making.

VI. CONFIDENTIAL INFORMATION

Confidential information belongs to the health services organization. Use of it by administrators, their business associates, friends or relatives for their own gain is a violation of the Code of Ethics and misuse of corporate property.

The interests of the organization are primary and insider information may not be used for personal gain. Its use may be interpreted as improper even though there is no monetary loss to the corporation.

APPENDIX I

American College of Healthcare Executives
Grievance Procedure

1. To be processed, a complaint must be filed in writing to the Committee on Ethics of the College within three years of the date of the alleged incident; and, the committee has the responsibility to look into incidents brought to its attention regardless of the informality of the information, provided the information can be documented or may be a matter of public record.

2. A copy of the complaint must be sent to the respondent, preferably by certified mail, by the staff of the College.

3. Upon receipt of the complaint, the Committee on Ethics shall refer the matter to the Regent of the area in which the respondent presently is employed. The Regent shall make inquiry into the matter and in the process the respondent shall be given an opportunity to be heard.

4. Upon completion of the inquiry the Regent shall present a complete report in writing to the Committee on Ethics. In the report, the Regent may make recommendations regarding the disposition of the case.

5. Upon receipt of the Regent's report, and following the Committee's review and action, a copy of the report shall be sent promptly to the respondent.

6. If the respondent wishes to appeal, he may do so formally by a written request. This request must be filed with the Committee within sixty days from the date of the Regent's report.

7. If a respondent so requests, or if the Committee on Ethics or the complainant wishes to pursue the matter further, then the Committee on Ethics shall recommend

to the ACHE Chairman the appointment of an ad hoc committee to hear the matter.

8. This ad hoc committee shall consist of three Fellows from the region of the respondent's area of employment at the time of the alleged infraction of the Code of Ethics. Adequate notice of the formation of this committee, notice of the hearing date, with an opportunity for representation, shall be mailed to the respondent. Notice of the ad hoc committee and the date of the hearing shall be given to the complainant. At least thirty days notice of the hearing date shall be given to all parties concerned. Reasonable requests for postponement shall be given consideration.

9. The ad hoc committee shall give the complainant and respondent adequate opportunity to present their cases and to be represented, if they so desire. At the close of the hearing, the ad hoc committee shall write a detailed report with recommendations to the Committee on Ethics.

10. A copy of this report shall go promptly to the respondent. If the respondent wishes to pursue the matter further, he may request, within sixty days of the date of the ad hoc committee's report, an appearance before the Committee on Ethics. The Committee shall give the respondent opportunity to state his case. Following this appeals hearing, the Committee on Ethics shall make its decision and provide the respondent with a copy of its report to the Board of Governors.

11. If the respondent wishes to pursue the matter further, he may request, within sixty days of the date of the Committee on Ethics report, a review of the case by the Board of Governors. Following a review by the Board of Governors, the Board shall make its decision and provide the respondent and complainant with a copy of its decision. The decision of the Board of Governors shall be final.

APPENDIX II

American Hospital Association

Guidelines on Ethical Conduct and Relationships for Health Care Institutions*

Health care institutions are service organizations that provide patient care and a varying range of education, research, public health, and social services for their communities. These institutions carry public responsibilities for their own conduct, the well-being of their patients, and the health of their communities. This role places special obligations upon health care institutions and their representatives to adhere to ethical principles of conduct. The following guidelines are intended to assist members of the American Hospital Association in defining their institutional policies, ethical relationships, and practices.

1. Good health is of utmost importance to the nation, to the community, and to every individual. Health care institutions should be interested in the overall health status of people in addition to providing direct patient care services.

2. The public has accorded high priority to the availability of services to the sick and injured, but there are limits to the individual and collective resources available for this purpose. Recognizing this, health care institutions should:

   a. Support the most effective use of economic and other resources to ensure access to comprehensive services of high quality.

   b. Deliver services efficiently.

3. The community's health objectives are advanced when all health care providers and social, welfare, educational, and other agencies work together in planning and offering improved services. Health care institutions should promote and support cooperation among each other, all providers, and community agencies in efforts to increase the results they could achieve separately.

4. Patient care services are inherently personal in nature. Health care institutions should maintain organizational relationships, policies, and systems that produce an environment that is conducive to humane and individualized care for those being served.

5. Individual religious and social beliefs and customs are important to each person. Health care institutions should, wherever possible and consistent with ethical commitments of the institution, ensure respect and consideration for the dignity and individuality of patients, employees, physicians, and others.

6. Health care institutions should establish and maintain internal policies, practices, standards of performance, and systematic methods of evaluation that emphasize high quality, safety, and effectiveness of care.

7. Health care institutions, being dependent upon community confidence and support, should accept an ethical sense of public accountability; reflect fairness, honesty, and impartiality in all activities and relationships; manage their resources prudently; and ensure that reports to the public are factual and clear in interpreting institutional goals, status, and accomplishments.

8. Health care institutions should relate to their communities and to each other constructively and in ways that merit and preserve public con-

fidence in them, both individually and collectively.

*Approved by the Board of Trustees of the American Hospital
Association, April 1, 1974.

SELECTED BIBLIOGRAPHY

"American Association of Occupational Health Nurses Code
of Ethics." *Occupational Health Nursing* 25(3):28,
March 1977.

"AMRA bylaws and code of ethics." American Medical Records
Association. *Medical Record News* 48(1):41-48, February
1977.

"A proposal for an ethics committee." American Academy
of Pediatrics. Reprinted in: *Hastings Center Report*
13(6):6-7, December 1983.

"Basic curriculum goals in medical ethics." [Special Re-
port] *New England Journal of Medicine* 312(4):253-
256.

"Code of ethics." *American Corrective Therapy Journal*
29(1):28, January/February 1975.

"Code of ethics." American Health Care Association. *Journal of the American Health Care Association* 2(2):19,
March 1976.

"Code of ethics." Revised 1977, The First District Dental
Society of New York. *New York Journal of Dentistry*
48(3):71-78, March 1978.

"Compensating for research injuries: the ethical and legal
implications of programs to redress injured subjects."
Washington, D.C.: U.S. Government Printing Office,
1982.

"Ethical issues in health care management." Proceedings
of the Seventeenth Annual Symposium on Hospital Affairs. Chicago, Ill.: University of Chicago, Graduate
Program in Hospital Administration, 1975.

"Ethics in the care of the elderly." *Quarterly, A Journal
of Long Term Care* 21(4):10-13, January 1986.

"Ethics in care provision: a specific example." *Quarterly, A Journal of Long Term Care* 21(4):14-16, January 1986.

"Guidelines: hospital committees on biomedical ethics." Chicago, Ill.: American Hospital Association 1984.

"Guidelines on ethical conduct and relationships for health care institutions." *Frontiers of Health Services Management* 1(1), September 1984.

"Hospital management corporations: creeping proprietarization." *Consumer Health Perspectives* 5(2):1-8, June 1978.

"How can medical-moral committees function effectively in Catholic health facilities?" *Hospital Progress* 64(4):77-78, April 1983.

"Implementing human research regulations: the adequacy and uniformity of federal rules and their implementation." Washington, D.C.: U.S. Government Printing Office, 1983.

"Institutional ethics committees. 'Recommended' now, but perhaps mandatory in the near future." *Cost Containment* 6(5):3-6, March 1984.

"It's a question of ethics." *Hospitals* 53 (23):86-88, December 1979.

"Maintaining ethical principles and surviving in a competitive environment." *Bulletin of the American Protestant Hospital Association* 47(2):9-13, 37, Fall 1983.

"Making health care decisions: the ethical and legal implications of informed consent in the patient-practitioner relationship." Washington, D.C.: U.S. Government Printing Office, 1982.

"Preserving a caring tradition." *Hospitals* September 1, 1983.

"The price of life: ethics and economics." *Report of the Minnesota Coalition on Health Care Costs*, December 1984.

"Screening and counseling, and education programs." Washington, D.C.: U.S. Government Printing Office, 1983.

"Securing access to health care: the ethical implications of differences in availability of health services." Washington, D.C.: U.S. Government Printing Office, 1983.

"Splicing life: the social and ethical issues of genetic engineering with human beings." Washington, D.C.: U.S. Government Printing Office, 1982.

"Suppliers, hospitals told to disclose common bonds." *Medical Products Salesman* 10(10):26, October 1979.

"Survey on institutional ethics committees." *National Society of Patient Representatives, Data Report.* Chicago, Ill.: American Hospital Association, August 1983.

"Way to reduce high cost of dying eludes health care professionals." *The Citizen* (Ottawa), May 7, 1986, p. 14.

Abram, M. B. "Ethical issues in health administration." *AUPHA Program Notes*, July/August 1981, pp. 8-14.

Ahern, Mary Layne. "Biomedical ethics committees confront prickly issues." *Hospitals* 58(15), August 1, 1984.

Ahern, Mary Layne. "How ethics committees can safely navigate untested legal waters." *Trustee* 37:10, October 1984.

Almquist, David D. "Code of ethics." *American Journal of Hospital Pharmacy* 37(2):185, February 1980.

Alper, Philip R. "The new language of hospital management."
New England Journal of Medicine 311(19):1249-1251,
November 8, 1984.

American College of Hospital Administrators Commission
on Ethics. *Code of Ethics*. Chicago, Ill.: American
College of Hospital Administrators, 1974.

American Hospital Association. *A Patient's Bill of Rights*.
Chicago, Ill.: American Hospital Association, 1972.

Annas, George J. "Ethics committees in neonatal care: substantive protection or procedural diversion?" *American
Journal of Public Health* 74(8):843-845, August 1984.

Appell, G. N. "Teaching anthropological ethics: developing
skills on ethical decision making and the nature of
moral education." *Anthropological Quarterly* 49(2):81-
88, April 1976.

Appley, Lawrence A. *Values in Management*. American Management Association, 1968.

Aroskar, Mila A. "Anatomy of an ethical dilemma: the practice." *American Journal of Nursing*, April 1980, p.
661-663.

Ashley, Benedict M., and Kevin D. O'Rourke. *Health Care
Ethics: A Theological Analysis*, 2nd edition. St.
Louis, Mo.: The Catholic Health Association of the
U.S., 1982.

Austin, Charles J. "What is health administration?" *Hospital Administration* 19(3):14-29, September 1974.

Avard, Denise, Glenn Griener and Jim Langstaff. "Hospital
ethics committees: survey reveals characteristics." *Dimensions of Health Services* 62(2):24-
26, February 1985.

Ayers, Stephen M. "When values compete: ethics committees and consensus." *Health Progress* 65(11), December 1984.

Bacon, Ernest. "Ethical conduct in the measure of excellence: how to survive in the eighties." *Hospital and Health Services Administration*, March/April 1983.

Bader, "Ethics: boards address issues beyond allocation of resources." *Trustee* 35(10), October 1982.

Bailey, Mary Ann. "Rationing and American health policy." *Journal of Health Politics, Policy and Law* 9(3), Fall 1984.

Baird, Charles W. *Advertising by Professionals*. Ottawa, Ill.: Green Hill Publishers, 1977.

Barkun, Harvey. "Ethical issues inherent in the choices of priorities - a case study." International Seminar for Administrators, King's Fund College, June 14, 1983.

Barry, John. "Law and health care." Canadian College of Health Record Administrators Conference, June 5, 1985.

Barry, Vincent. *Moral Issues in Business*. Belmont, Calif.: Wadsworth Publishing Company, 1979.

Bates, David V. "Are ethics of industry appropriate to medical care?" *Hospital Trustee* 3(3):11-14, September/October 1979.

Bauer, R. and D. Finn. "What is a corporate social audit?" *Harvard Business Review*, January-February 1973, p.37-48.

Bayer, Ronald, et al. "The care of the terminally ill: morality and economics." *New England Journal of Medicine* 309(24):1490-1494, December 15, 1983.

Bayer, Ronald, Arthur L. Caplan and Norman Daniels. *In Search of Equity*. New York: Plenum Press, 1983.

Beauchamp, Tom L., and Norman E. Bowie, editors. *Ethical Theory and Business*. Englewood Cliffs, N.J.: Prentice-Hall, Inc., 1979.

Berger, J. D. "The ethical side of advertising." *Hospital Forum* 24(6):35, 38-39, November/December 1981.

Bergman, A. B. "Needed: humanism in health program managers." *Journal of Health Politics, Policy and Law* 3(3):298-302, Fall 1978.

Binder, Jim. "Value conflicts in health care organizations." *Nursing Economics* 1(2):114-119, September/October 1983.

Blandford, John M. "Ethical considerations inherent in choices on priorities." International Seminar for Administrators, King's Fund College, June 14, 1983.

Bondurant, S. "Some reflections on the relationships between universities and industry as they influence the evolution of the medical-industrial complex." *NC Medical Journal* 45(4):235-236, April 1984.

Boyd, K. M., editor. *The Ethics of Resource Allocation in Health Care*. Edinburgh, Scotland: Edinburgh University Press, 1979.

Brenner, Steven N., and Earl A. Molander. "Is the ethics of business changing?" *Harvard Business Review* January/February 1977.

Brodeur, Dennis. "Toward a clear definition of ethics committees." *Linacre Quarterly* 51(3):233-247, August 1984.

Bromberg, M. D. "Economics, ethics and access: the perspective of investor-owned hospitals." *National Forum Hospital Health Affairs*, 1983, p. 83-93.

Brown, Montague. "Contract management: legal and policy implications." *Inquiry* 18(1):8-17, Spring 1981.

Brown, Peter G. "Ethics and public policy: a preliminary agenda." *Policy Studies Journal* 7(1):132-137, Autumn 1978.

Brozovich, John P. "Managing change through values." *Healthcare Executive* 1(3):45-47, March/April 1986.

Burns, Chester R., editor. *Legacies in Ethics and Medicine*. New York: Science History Publications, 1977.

Callahan, Daniel. "Applied ethics: a strategy for fostering professional responsibility." *Carnegie Quarterly* Spring/Summer 1980.

Callahan, Daniel. "Health and society: some ethical imperatives." *Daedalus* 106:22-23, Winter 1977.

Callahan, Daniel. "Obligations of hospital trustees." *Hastings Center Report* 72(6):4, December 1982.

Callahan, Daniel, and Sissela Bok. *Ethics Teaching in Higher Education*. New York: Plenum Press, c1980.

Camenisch, Paul F. "Business ethics: on getting to the heart of the matter." *Business and Professional Ethics Journal* 1(1):59-69, Fall 1981.

Campbell, Alister V. *Medicine, Health and Justice: The Problem of Priorities*. Edinburgh, Scotland: Churchill Livingstone, 1978.

Campbell, J. D., and K. McEwin. "The hospital ethics committee." *Medical Journal of Australia* 1(4):68-69, February 21, 1981.

Canadian College of Health Service Executives. *Code of Ethics*. Ottawa, Ontario, 1979.

Canadian Health Record Association. *Code of Practice*. Oshawa, Ontario, June 5, 1978.

Canadian Health Record Association. *Guidelines to the Code of Practice*. Oshawa, Ontario, May 1980.

Canadian Hospital Council. *Hospital Ethics: A Code*. Toronto, Ontario, 1941.

Canadian Medical Association. *Code of Ethics*. Ottawa, Ontario, June 1977.

Canadian Nurses Association. *Code of Ethics for Nursing*. Ottawa, Ontario, February 1985.

Chandler, Ralph C. "Ethics and public policy." *Commonwealth* 105(10):302-306, May 12, 1978.

Chown, Ed. "Ethical decisions: no simple recipe." *Hospital Trustee* 10(1):4, January/February 1986.

Chown, Ed. "Commentary." (on Levey and Hill) *Journal of Health Administration Education* 4(2):240-243, Spring 1986.

Christie, Joel R. "Towards excellence in decision making." *Health Management Forum* 7(2):38-46, Summer 1986.

Clark, Arva Rosenfeld, Alan Sheldon and Curtis P. McLaughlin. "Policy-making, medical ethics, and health institutions: the roles of physician and manager." *Ethics in Science and Medicine* 3(3):165-178, September 1976.

Cohen, Cynthia. "Interdisciplinary consultation in the care of the critically ill and dying: the role of one hospital ethics committee." *Critical Care Medicine* 10(11):776-784, November 1982.

College of Nurses of Ontario. *Guidelines for Ethical Behaviour in Nursing*. Toronto, Ontario, September 1980.

Cooper, Terry L. *The Responsible Administrator: An Approach to Ethics for the Administrative Role*. Port Washington, N.Y.: Associated Faculty Press, 1982.

Countryman, Kathleen M., and Alexandra B. Gelas. "Development and implementation of a patient's bill of rights in hospitals." Chicago, Ill.: American Hospital Association, 1980.

Cranford, R. E., et al. "The emergence of institutional ethics committees." *Law, Medicine and Health Care* 12(1):13-20, February 1984.

Cranford, Ronald E., and A. Edward Doudera, editors. *Institutional Ethics Committees and Health Care*. Ann Arbor, Mich.: AUPHA Press, 1984.

Cunico, E. "Health care values redefined." *Hospital Manager* 15(1):3, January/February 1985.

Cunningham, Robert M., Jr. "Changing philosophies in medical care and the rise of the investor-owned hospital." *New England Journal of Medicine* 307(13):817-819, September 23, 1982.

Cunningham, Robert M., Jr. *The Healing Mission and the Business Ethic*. Chicago, Ill.: Pluribus Press, 1982.

Cunningham, Robert M., Jr. "More than a business: are hospitals forgetting their basic mission?" *Hospitals* 57(2), January 16, 1983.

Darr, Kurt. "Administrative ethics and the health services manager." *Hospital and Health Services Administration* 29(2):120-136, March/April 1984.

Darr, Kurt. *Case Studies in Health Administration*, Volume 4, Ethics for Health Services Managers. Chicago, Ill.: Foundation of the American College of Healthcare Executives, 1985.

Darr, Kurt. "The ethical imperative in health services governance and management." *Hospital and Health Services Administration* 31(2):53-66, March/April 1986.

Davis, Dona S. "Nursing: an ethic of caring." *Humane Medicine* 2(1):19-25, May 1986.

Davis, Michael. "Conflict of interest." *Business and Professional Ethics Journal* 1(4):17-27, Summer 1982.

Dearden, Robert W. "Can there be social justice from a health system?" International Seminar for Administrators, King's Fund College, June 14, 1983.

DeGeorge, Richard T. "The moral responsibility of the hospital." *Journal of Medicine and Philosophy* 7(1):87-100, February 1982.

DeGeorge, Richard T., and Joseph A. Pichler, editors. *Ethics, Free Enterprise, and Public Policy*. New York: Oxford University Press, 1978.

Dhawan, K. C., and Ursula Tokateloff. "Attitudes toward ethics: a survey of Canadian top business executives." Monograph, December 1975.

Dobbin, Lucy C. "Ethics and leadership day to day." CCHSE National Conference, June 17, 1986 (cassette).

Dolan, Thomas C. "Six challenges for the future." (Invited Essay given at the 1984 AUPHA Annual Meeting, April 26-29, Washington, D.C.) *Journal of Health Administration Education* 2(3):281-289, Summer 1984.

Donaldson, L. J. "Care of the elderly in hospitals and homes: foci of discontent." *Journal of the Royal Society for Health* 103(5):181-185, October 1983.

Donaldson, Thomas and Patricia H. Weshane, editors. *Ethical Issues in Business: A Philosophical Approach*. Englewood Cliffs, N.J.: Prentice-Hall, Inc. 1979.

Doucet, Herbert. "Ethics in a high tech world." *CHAC Review* 12(4):18-20, Winter 1984.

Doucet, Herbert. "Ethics committees: protection for patients." *Hospital Trustee* 9(5):27-29, September/October 1985.

Doudera, A. Edward, and J. Douglas Peters, editors. *Legal and Ethical Aspects of Treating Critically and Terminally Ill Patients*. Ann Arbor, Mich.: AUPHA Press, 1982.

Emerton, E. "Spotting scams; preventing kickbacks." *Dimensions in Health Service* 58(10):16-18, October 1981.

Ertel, P. Y., et al. "Ethical and operational issues concerning DRGs and the prospective payment system." *Topics in Health Record Management* 4(3):10-31, March 1984.

Esqueda, Kathi. "Hospital ethics committees: four case studies." *Hospital Medical Staff* 7(11):26-30, November 1978.

Evans, Tom. "Accountability for ethical and value judgments in the management of health organizations." International Seminar for Administrators, King's Fund College, June 16, 1983.

Ewell, Charles M., Jr. "Conflict of interest?" *Osteopathic Hospitals* October 1979.

Fajardo, Ortiz G. "The role of the hospital in a changing world." *World Hospital* 15(3):165-169, August 1979.

Ferguson, Cherry G. "Medical ethical issues: are you addressing them?" *Dimensions in Health Service* 61(8):30-31, 33, 25, August 1984.

Ferland, J. "Outline of a moral policy on the care of the dying in hospital surroundings." *Catholic Hospital* 7(1):16-18, January/February 1979.

Fishkin, James. "Moral principles and public policy." *Daedalus* 108(4):55-67, Autumn 1979.

147

Fleischman, Alan R., and Thomas H. Murray. "Ethics committees for Infant Doe?" *Hastings Center Report* 13 (6):5-9, December 1983.

Frankena, William K. *Ethics*, 2nd edition. Englewood Cliffs, N.J.: Prentice-Hall, 1973.

Freedman, Benjamin. "One philosopher's experience on an ethics committee." *Hastings Center Report* 11(2):20-22, April 1981.

Freedman, Benjamin. "Ethics and allocation: the business of health care is not a business." CCHSE National Conference, June 15, 1986 (cassette).

Freedman, David, H. "Ethics: who decides right from wrong?" *Infosystems* 30(8):34-36, August 1983.

Freidson, Eliot, editor. *The Hospital in Modern Society*. New York: Free Press of Glencoe, 1963.

French, Peter A. "Collective responsibility and the practice of medicine." *Journal of Medicine and Philosophy* 7(1):65-85, February 1982.

Friedman, Emily. "Health care resource allocation: the trustee's role." Chaiker Abbis Forum on Hospital Governance, July 31, 1986, Toronto, Ontario.

Friedman, Emily. "Rationing and the identified life." *Hospital Medical Staff* 13(5):10-17, May 1984.

Friedman, Emily. "Trying to balance reality and ethics." *Hospitals* 58(18):91-97, September 16, 1984.

Fritzsche, David J., and Helmut Becker. "Linking management behavior to ethical philosophy - an empirical investigation." *Academy of Management Journal* 27(1):166-175, January 1984.

Fuchs, Victor R. *Who Shall Live? Health, Economics, and Social Choice*. New York: Basic Books, 1974.

Ganos, Doreen, et al., editors. *Difficult Decisions in Medical Ethics*. Volume 4, 1981-1982.

Gilmore, Anne. "Access to health care: how can costs be contained?" *Canadian Medical Association Journal* 130(5):614, 616-618, March 1, 1984.

Glazer, Myron. "Ten whistleblowers and how they fared." *Hastings Center Report* 13(6):33-41, December 1983.

Goldman, Alan H. "Business ethics: profits, utilities, and moral rights." *Philosophy and Public Affairs* 9(3):260-286, Spring 1980.

Goldsmith, Seth B. *Health Care Management: A Contemporary Perspective*. Rockville, Md.: Aspen Systems Corp., 1981.

Goodpaster, K. E., and J. B. Matthews. "Can a corporation have a conscience?" *Harvard Business Review*, January/February 1982, p. 132-141.

Gray, Bradford H., editor. *The New Health Care For Profit: Doctors and Hospitals in a Competitive Environment*. Washington, D.C.: National Academy Press, 1983.

Greenfield, Harry I. *Accountability in Health Facilities*. New York: Praeger Publishers, 1975.

Gregory, Charles L. "Ethics: a management tool? A profile of the values of hospital administrators." *Hospital and Health Services Administration* 29(2):102-119, March/April 1984.

Griffith, John R. "The proper way to live: remarks on the teaching of hospital administration." *Journal of Health Administration Education* 1(1):27-36, Winter 1983.

Guidelines on the Ethical Conduct and Relationships for Health Care Institutions. Chicago, Ill.: American Hospital Association, April 1, 1974.

Guidi, Doris Jordan. *Hospital Ethics Committees: Potential Mediators for Educational and Policy Change*. Ann Arbor, Mich.: University Microfilms International, 1983.

Harrison, Colin P. "Code of ethics." *Canadian Medical Association Journal* 119(2):117-118, July 1978.

Harrison, Fernande P. "Consider values-based management." *Health Management Forum* 6(3):4-17, Autumn 1985.

Hayes, Thomas J. "Ethics in business: problem identification and potential solutions." *Hospital Material Management Quarterly* 4(4):35-42, May 1983.

Hiller, Marc D. *Medical Ethics and the Law: Implications for Public Policy*. Cambridge, Mass.: Ballinger Publishing Company, 1981.

Hiller, Marc D. "Ethics and health care administration: issues in education and practice." *Journal of Health Administration Education* 2(2):147-192, Spring 1984.

Hofman, Paul B. "Upholding patient rights through ethical policymaking." *Trustee* 38(4):15-16, April 1985.

Hofman, Paul B. "Providing an institutional framework for resolving ethical dilemmas." *Health Management Quarterly*, Winter 1984-1985, p. 12-13.

Hosford, Bowen. *Bioethics Committees*. Rockville, Md.: Aspen Systems Corporation, 1986.

Howe, Elizabeth, and Jerome Kaufman. "Ethics and professional practice in planning and related policy professions." *Policy Studies Journal* 9(4, Special Issue #2):585-595, 1980-1981.

Hull, Richard T. "Defining nursing ethics apart from medical ethics." *Kansas Nurse* 55(8):5, September 1980.

150

Hull, Richard T. "The function of professional codes of ethics." *Westminster Institute Review* 1(3):12-13, October 1981.

Johnson, Richard L. "The day after." *Hospital and Health Services Administration* 30(6):106-117, November/December.

Johnson, Spencer C. "The public interest in an era of competition." Wagner Memorial Lecture. Ithaca, N.Y.: Cornell University, May 9, 1986.

Kahn, Lynn. "Ethical issues dominate hospital leadership forum." *The Hospital Medical Staff* 13(10) October 1984.

Kalchbrenner, J., M. J. Kelly and D. G. McCarthy. "Ethics committees and ethicists in Catholic hospitals." *Hospital Progress* 64(9):47-51, September 1983.

Kapp, M. B. "Legal and ethical implications of health care reimbursement by diagnosis-related groups." *Law, Medicine and Health Care* 12(6):245-253, 278, December 1984.

Kaufman, Jerome L. "Ethics and planning: some insights from the outside." [Book Reviews] *Journal of the American Planning Association* 47(2):196-199, April 1981.

Kavanagh, John P. "The sinking of sun ship: a case study in managerial ethics." *Business and Professional Ethics Journal* 1(4):1-13, Summer 1982.

King, Lester S. "The AMA gets a new code of ethics." *Journal of the American Medical Association* 249(10):1338-1342, March 11, 1983.

Kinzer, David M. "Commentary." (on Levey and Hill) *Journal of Health Administration Education* 4(2):244-248, Spring 1986.

Knight, Edward H., and Jannice E. Moore. *To Be or Not to Be - Involved*. Edmonton, Alberta: Alberta Hospital Association, 1983.

Knight, James A. "The essence of ethical codes and oaths." [Editorial] *Journal of Clinical Psychiatry* 42(6):222-223, June 1981.

Knowles, John H., editor. *Hospitals, Doctors, and the Public Interest*. Cambridge, Mass.: Harvard University Press, 1965.

Kuperberg, J. R. "Ethics, accountability and decision making." *Journal of Long-Term Care Administration* 6(3): 25-34, 1978.

L'Association des directeurs generaux des services de sante et des services sociaux du Quebec. *Regles d'Ethique*, Montreal, Avril 1978.

Lane, G. Alan. "On medical morals and ethics." *Health Management Forum* 4(3):60-71, Autumn 1983.

Langholm, O., and J. Lunde. "Empirical methods for business ethics research." *Review of Social Economy* 35(2):133-142, October 1977.

Last, John M. "Some ethical issues in public health." *Canadian Journal of Public Health* 77(2):75, 77, March/April 1986.

Last, John M. "Individual privacy and health information: an ethical dilemma?" *Canadian Journal of Public Health* 77(3):168-169, May/June 1986.

Levey, Samuel, and James Hill. "Between survival and social responsibility: in Search of an Ethical Balance." *Journal of Health Administration Education* 4(2):225-231, Spring 1986.

Levine, Carol. "Ethics and health cost containment." *Hastings Center Report* 9(1):10-13, February 1971.

Levine, Carol. "Hospital ethics committees: a guarded prognosis." *Hastings Center Report* 7(3):25-27, June 1977.

Levine, Carol. "Questions and (some very tentative) answers about hospital ethics committees." *Hastings Center Report* 14(3):9-12, June 1984.

Levinson, Harry. "The changing role of the hospital administrator." *Health Care Management Review* 1(1):79-89, Winter 1979.

Luft, Harold S. "Health maintenance organization and the rationing of medical care." *Milbank Memorial Fund Quarterly* 60(2):268-306, Spring 1982.

Maccoby, Michael. "The corporate climber has to find his heart." *Fortune*, December 1976, p. 98-104.

MacDonald, Mary Susan. *The Feasibility of Developing a Code of Ethics for Canadian Health Administrators* (thesis), Toronto, Ontario: University of Toronto, September 1977.

MacDonald, Mary S. "Does health administration represent a new form of professionalism?" *Health Management Forum*, Winter 1982, p. 10-18.

Mackenzie, Norah. *The Professional Ethic and the Hospital Service*. London, England: English University Press, 1971.

MacNeil, H. "The board's mandate--operating the hospital." *Hospital Trustee* 7(3):16-18, May/June 1983.

MacStravic, R. E. S. "Market positioning: customer and product mix." *Health Care Planning and Marketing* 1(3):47-56, October 1981.

MacStravic, R. E. S. "Persuasive communication strategies for hospitals." *Health Care Management Review* 9(2):69-75, Spring 1984.

Mailick, Mildred D., and Helen Rehr, editors. *In the Patient's Interest: Access to Hospital Care*. New York: PRODIST, 1981.

Mamana, John P. "Ethics and technology: crossroads in decision making." *Trustee* 35(1):33, 36, 38, January 1982.

Marty, Martin E. "Financial retrenchment in the health sciences and ethical implications for management." *Journal of Health Administration Education* 3(2):103-111, Spring 1985, part II.

Maxwell, Robert J. "Commentary." (on Levey and Hill) *Journal of Health Administration Education* 4(2):232-234, Spring 1986.

May, W. "Professionals, administrators and hospitals: moral conflicts." *NAPPH Journal* 11(4):38-44.

McConnell, Terrance C. *Moral Issues in Health Care: An Introduction to Medical Ethics*. Belmont, Calif.: Wadsworth Inc., 1982.

McCullough, Laurence B. "Moral dilemmas and economic realities." *Hospital and Health Services Administration* 30(5):63-75, September/October 1985.

McElhenny, Thomas K., editor. *Medical Ethics--Study and Teaching--United States*, 3rd edition. Philadelphia, Pa.: Society for Health and Human Values, 1976.

McGeorge, Ken. "A call for moral leadership in health services administration." *Health Management Forum* 1(1): 27-31, Spring 1980.

McNerney, Walter J. "Managing ethical dilemmas." *Journal of Health Administration Education* 3(3):331-340, Summer 1985.

Mechanic, David. "The transformation of health providers." *Health Affairs* (Millwood) 3(1), Spring 1984.

Menzel, Paul T. *Medical Costs, Moral Choices, A Philosophy of Health Care Economics in America*. New Haven, Conn.: Yale University Press, 1983.

Meyer, Chuck. "Sin boldly: ethical issues of DRGs." *Hospital and Health Services Administration* 31(3):83-90, May/June 1986.

Michelman, J. H. "Some ethical consequences of economic competition." *Journal of Business Ethics* 2:79-87, 1983.

Miklos, E. "Ethical aspects of administrative action: implications for research and preparation." In *Administrator's Notebook* 26(5):2, Chicago, Ill.: University of Chicago, 1978.

Mintzberg, H. "The case for corporate social responsibility." *Journal of Business Strategy* 4(2):3-15, Fall 1983.

Monagle, J. F. "Bioethicist on hospital association staff sees upsurge in medical ethics problems." [Interview] *Review-Federation of American Hospitals* 16(6):40-41, November/December 1983.

Monagle, J. F. "Blueprints for hospital ethics committees." *California Hospital Association Insight* 8(20):1-4, June 26, 1984.

Mondragon, Fred E. "Public accountability and human services orientation." *Education for Health Administration*, Vol. II. Ann Arbor, Mich.: Health Administration Press, 1975, p. 185-197.

Mooney, Mary Margaret. "The code for nurses: a survey of its content, constitutive structure, and usefulness to the nursing profession." *Oklahoma Nurse* 25(5):11, June 1980.

Munson, Ronald. *Intervention and Reflection: Basic Issues in Medical Ethics*. Belmont, Calif.: Wadsworth Publishing Company, Inc., 1983.

Nash, Laura L. "Ethics without the sermon." *Harvard Business Review* 59(6):79-90, November/December 1981.

Neuhauser, D. "Ethics in hospital and health administration." *Health Matrix* 2(2):49-53, Summer 1984.

Newton, Lisa H. "Lawgiving for professional life: reflections on the place of the professional code." *Business and Professional Ethics Journal* 1(1):41-53, Fall 1981.

Newton, Lisa H. "Collective responsibility in health care." *Journal of Medicine and Philosophy* 7(1):11-21, February 1982.

Nutter, D. O. "Access to care and the evolution of corporate, for-profit medicine." *New England Journal of Medicine* 311(14):917-919, October 4, 1984.

Oglesby, D. Kirk, Jr. "Ethics and hospital administration." *Hospital and Health Services Administration* 30(5):29-43, September/October 1985.

O'Rourke, K. "An ethical perspective on investor-owned medical care corporations." *Frontier Health Services Management* 1(1):10-26, September 1984.

O'Sullivan, Michael J. "Ethics and health planning: implications for education." *Health Policy and Education* 2(2):103-117, September 1981.

Paigen, Beverly. "Controversy at Love Canal." *Hastings Center Report* 12(3):29-37, June 1982.

Pellegrino, Edmund D. "Catholic hospitals: survival without moral compromise." *Health Progress* 66(4):42-49, May 1985.

Pellegrino, Edmund D. "The ethics of collective judgments in medicine and health care." [Editorial] *Journal of Medicine and Philosophy* 7(1):3-10, February 1982.

Pellegrino, Edmund D. "What is a profession?" *Journal of Allied Health* 12(3):168-176, August 1983.

Pence, Gregory E. *Ethical Options in Medicine*. Oradell, N.J.: Medical Economics Company, 1980.

Pence, Terry. *Ethics in Nursing: An Annotated Bibliography*. New York: National League for Nursing, 1983.

Peters, Joseph P., and Ronald C. Wacker. "Strategic planning: hospital strategic planning must be rooted in values and ethics." *Hospitals* 56(12) June 16, 1982.

Peters, Joseph P., and Ronald C. Wacker. "Reconciling ethical and marketplace values in service program design." *Trustee* 35(12):30-40, 43, December 1982.

Pichler, Joseph A., Elliott Lehman and Eric Madr. "The liberty principle: a basis for management ethics." *Business and Professional Ethics* 2(2):19, 38, Winter 1983.

Powers, Charles W. *Ethics in the Education of Business Managers*. Hastings-on-Hudson, N.Y.: Hastings Center, 1980.

Powers, C. W., and D. Vogel. "Ethics in the education of business managers." *Institute of Society, Ethics, and the Life Sciences*, 1980, p. 3.

President's Commission for the Study of Ethical Problems in Medicine and Biomedical and Behavioral Research. "Defining Death: Medical, Legal and Ethical Issues in the Determination of Death." Washington, D.C.: U.S. Government Printing Office, July 1981.

Preston, T. A. "The artificial heart controversy: research, rationing, and regulation." *Medical World News* 26(3): 37, February 11, 1985.

Purtilo, Ruth B. "Ethics consultations in the hospital." *Sounding Board. New England Journal of Medicine* 311:15, October 11, 1984.

Purtilo, Ruth B., and Christine K. Cassel. *Ethical Dimensions in the Health Professions.* Philadelphia, Pa.: W. B. Saunders, 1981.

Rakoff, Vivian. "The fatal question." *Health Management Forum* 6(3):67-76, Autumn 1985.

Ramsey, Paul. *The Patient as a Person; Explorations in Medical Ethics.* New Haven, Conn.: Yale University Press, 1970.

Randal, Judith. "Are ethics committees alive and well?" *Hastings Center Report* 13(6):10-12, December 1983.

Read, William. "Ethical dilemmas in a changing health care environment: hospital ethics committees." *Health Research and Educational Trust*, 1983, p. 1-6.

Rehr, Helen, editor. *Ethical Dilemmas in Health Care: A Professional Search for Solutions.* Published for the Doris Seigal Memorial Fund of the Mount Sinai Medical Center by PRODIST, 1978.

Relman, A. S. "The new medical-industrial complex." *New England Journal of Medicine* 303:963-970, 1980.

Relman, A. S. "Investor-owned hospitals and health care costs." *New England Journal of Medicine* 309:370-372, 1983.

Relman, A. S., J. Bedrosian and R. J. Reitemeier. "The medical-industrial complex: debate." *Urban Health* 13(6):30-36, 51, July 1984.

Relman, Arnold S. "Economic considerations in emergency care: what are hospitals for?" [Editorial] *New England Journal of Medicine* 312(6):372-373, February 7, 1985.

Reverby, S. "Stealing the golden eggs: Ernest Amory Codman and the science and management of medicine." *Bulletin of the History of Medicine* 55(2):156-171, Summer 1981.

Rich, Pat. "Good medicine crashes against financial reality." *The Medical Post*, March 18, 1986, p. 6.

Robb, J. Wesley. "Analysis of choice value conflict." *Journal of Long-Term Care Administration* 4(4):14-28, 1976.

Robb, J. Wesley. "The allocation of limited medical resources: an ethical perspective." *The Pharos Spring* 1981.

Roberts, John. "The moral character of management practice." *Journal of Management Studies* 21(3):287-302, July 1984.

Robertson, J. A. "Ethics committees in hospitals: alternative structures and responsibilities." *Connecticut Medicine* 48(7):975-976, July 1984.

Rogers, William R., and Davis Barnard, editors. *Nourishing the Humanistic in Medicine: Interactions With the Social Sciences*. Pittsburgh, Pa.: University of Pittsburgh Press, 1979.

Rosen, Bernard. *Ethics in the Undergraduate Curriculum*. New York: The Hastings Center, 1980.

Rozovsky, Lorne E. "Conflict of interest on hospital boards." *Hospital Trustee* 1(2):14-15, September/ October 1977.

Ruddick, W., and W. Finn. "Objections to hospital philosophers." *Journal of Medical Ethics* 11(1):42-46, March 1985.

Sauer, James E. "Ethical problems facing the healthcare industry." *Hospital and Health Services Administration* 30(5):44-53, September/October 1985.

Saward, Ernest, and Andrew Sorensen. "Competition, profit, and the HMO." *New England Journal of Medicine* 306(5): 929-931, April 15, 1982.

Schafer, A. "Moral leadership in health services." *Dimensions in Health Services* 56(11):37-40, November 1979.

Schwartz, Daniel H. "The patient's bill of rights and the hospital administrator." In *Bioethics and Human Rights* edited by E. L. and B. Bandman. Boston, Mass.: Little, Brown, and Company, 1978.

Secretary of State. *The Canadian Style: A Guide to Writing and Editing*. Toronto, Ontario: Dundurn Press, 1985.

Seiden, Dena J. "Ethics for hospital administrators." *Hospital and Health Services Administration* 28(2), March/April 1983.

Settlemyre, J. T. "Caring: putting patients first begins with management skills." *Hospital Forum* 27(3):48-50, 53, May/June 1984.

Shaw, Margery W. and A. Edward Doudera, editors. *Defining Human Life: Medical, Legal, and Ethical Implications*. Ann Arbor, Mich.: AUPHA Press, 1983.

Shea, Michael. "Ethical principles." *Health Services Management Intramural*, Ottawa, Ontario, May 9, 1986.

Sherman, S. R. "AMA judicial chairman sees emergence of hospital ethics panels as an inevitability." [Interview] *Review-Federation of American Hospitals* 16(6): 30, 32, November/December 1983.

Sherrard, Heather. *Institutional Ethics Committees: Recommendations for Action*. Ottawa, Ontario: Canadian Hospital Association, 1986.

Sherwin, Douglas S. "The ethical roots of the business system." *Harvard Business Review*, November/December 1983, p. 183-192.

Sherwood, Frank P. "Professional ethics." *Public Management* 57(6):13-14, June 1975.

Sims-Jones, Nicola. "Ethical dilemmas in the NICU." *Canadian Nurse/L'infirmiere canadienne* 82(4):24-26, April 1986.

Smith, C. Thomas, Jr. "A search for easy answers in complex circumstances." *Hospital and Health Services Administration* 30(5):54-62, September/October 1985.

Smith, S. Douglas. "Ethical entrepreneurship: a question of risk." *Healthcare Executive* 1(5):30-33, July/August 1986.

Smurl, James F. "Distributing the burden fairly: ethics and national health policy." *Man and Medicine* 5(2):97-125, 1980.

Smythe, S. "Hospital advertising--is it ethical?" *Texas Hospital* 39(3):12-14, August 1983.

Snedden, J. Douglas. "Ethical issues in the determination of program priorities." International Seminar for Administrators, King's Fund College, June 14, 1983.

Starkweather, David B. "Doing good or doing well, or so what?" *The Western Network of Note* 4:1-4, September 1983.

Starkweather, David B. "In search of social enterprise: a fable." *Hospital and Health Services Administration* 31(3):45-57, May/June 1986.

Sternberg, Steve. "Lying hopelessly ill, infant tests new law of hospital survival." [News] *Washington Post* April 3, 1983, p. A4.

Stevens, J. E. "Hospital ethics committees." *Quarterly Review Bulletin* 9(6):162-163, June 1983.

Storch, Janet L. "Moral and ethical obligations of health executives regarding patients' rights and advocacy." *Health Management Forum* 3(2):15-24, Summer 1982.

Storch, Janet L. "Commentary." (on Levey and Hill) *Journal of Health Administration Education* 4(2):238-239, Spring 1986.

Storch, Janet L. "Ethical issues in research: management responses." CCHSE National Conference, June 16, 1986 (cassette).

Storch, Janet, John Borthwick, David Schiff and Glenn Grenier. "Preparing health service managers for ethical decision making." CCHSE-CHA-AUPHA Colloquium, June 17, 1986 (cassette).

Stuart, Barbara K., and Carole Steele. "Can a hospital mean business?" *Healthcare Financial Management* 37 (12):26-28, December 1983.

Sturd, Jan. "Patient advocates: how managers can work with them." *Health Management Forum* 1:4, 50-62, Winter 1980.

Sufrin, Sidney C. "How moral can a business be?" *Christian Century* 100(6):186-188, March 2, 1983.

Summers, James W. "Doing good and doing well; ethics, professionalism and success." *Hospital and Health Services Administration* 29(2):85-100, March/April 1984.

Summers, James W. "Closing unprofitable services: ethical issues and management responses." *Hospital and Health Services Administration* 30(5):8-28, September/October 1985.

Swett, Jonathan N. "Reconstitution of the not-for-profit hospital: new ethics, new equity." *Hospital and Health Services Administration* 30(36):20-30, May/June 1985.

Tancredi, Laurence R. *Ethics for Health Care*. Washington, D.C.: National Academy of Sciences, 1974.

Text of AMA's new principles of ethics. *American Medical News* 23(30):9, August 8, 1980.

The Hastings Center's Bibliography of Ethics, Biomedicine, and Professional Responsibility. The Hastings Center. Frederick, Md.: University Publications of America in association with the Hastings Center, 1984.

The Teaching of Ethics in Higher Education: A Report. Hastings-on-Hudson, N.Y.: Hastings Center, Institute of Society, Ethics, and the Life Sciences, 1980.

Thomasma, David C. "Hospital's ethical responsibilities as technology, regulation grow." *Hospital Progress* 63(12):74-79, December 1982.

Thurow, Lester Carl. Sounding Board. "Learning to say no." *New England Journal of Medicine* 311(24):1569-1572, December 1984.

Tregunno, Deborah J. "Ethics and hospital administration: development of a questionnaire to assess awareness and influences." Major paper. Edmonton, Alberta: University of Alberta, 1985.

Tregunno, Deborah J. "Ethics and hospital administration." *Health Management Forum* 7(1):58-69, Spring 1986.

Tuggle, R. "Is advertising right?" [Editorial] *Hospital Forum* 19(7):16, December 1976.

Uhlmann, Richard F., Walter J. McDonald and Thomas S. Inui. "Epidemiology of no-code orders in an academic hospital." *Western Journal of Medicine* 140(1):114-116, January 1984.

Umbeck, P. F. "The church related hospital in a secular society." *Bulletin of the American Protestant Hospital Association* 41(1):14-15, 28-29, Spring 1977.

Usherwood, Bob. "Towards a code of professional ethics." *Aslib Proceedings* 33(6):233-242, June 1981.

Uustal, Diane B. "Values clarification in nursing: application to practice." *American Journal of Nursing* 78 (12):2058-2063, December 1978.

Values in Conflict: Ethical Issues in Hospital Care. Report of the Special Committee on Biomedical Ethics. American Hospital Association, February 1985.

Veatch, Robert M., and Roy Branson, editors. *Ethics and Health Policy.* Cambridge, Mass.: Ballinger Publishing, 1976.

Veatch, Robert M. "Hospital ethics committees: is there a role?" *Hastings Center Report* 7(3):22-25, June 1977.

Veatch, Robert M. "Professional medical ethics: the grounding of its principles." *The Journal of Medicine and Philosophy* 4(1):1-19, 1979.

Veatch, Robert M. *A Theory of Medical Ethics.* New York: Basic Books, 1981.

Walch, W. E., and S. Tseng. "Marketing: handle with care." *Trustee* 37(8):19-21, August 1984.

Walker, R. C. "Ethical dilemmas in the governance and management of hospitals." CCHSE National Conference, June 16, 1986 (cassette).

Wallace, C. "M.D.'s qualms about profit motive scuttle HCA's bid to buy Harvard-affiliated unit." [News] *Modern Health Care* 13(12):76, 78, December 1983.

Walton, Clarence Cyril. *Ethics and the Executive*. Prentice-Hall, 1969.

Walton, Clarence C. "Business ethics: the present and the future. A review of recent literature." *Hastings Center Report*, October 1980, p. 16-20.

Wasserman, Jeffrey, Joel J. May, Daniel H. Schwartz, and Joy Hinson Penticuff. "The doctor, the patient, and the DRG." [Case Study and Commentaries] *Hastings Center Report* 13(56):23-25, October 1983.

Weber, Leonard J. "Infant treatment decisions: ethics and cost." *Health Progress* 65(11), December 1984.

Wielk, Carol A. "Human experimentation: issues before the hospital administrator." *Hospital and Health Services Administration* 22(3):4-25, Summer 1977.

Wikler, D. I. "Persuasion and coercion for health: ethical issues in government efforts to change lifestyles." *Milbank Memorial Fund Quarterly* 56:303-338, Summer 1978.

Wikler, D. "Forming an ethical response to for-profit health care." *Business Health* 2(3):25-29, January/February 1985.

Williams, Kenneth J. "Hospitals." In Warren T. Reich, editor, *Encyclopedia of Bioethics*, Volume 2. New York: Free Press, 1978, p. 677-683.

Williams, Kenneth J. *Medical Care Quality and the Public Trust: A Corporate Guide for Hospital Trustees, Medical Staff, and Administrators*. Chicago, Ill.: Pluribus Press Inc., 1982.

Wilson, Robert N. "Commentary on business ethics: on getting to the heart of the matter." *Business and Professional Ethics Journal* 1(1):71-75, Fall 1981.

Winston, William E., and Albert J. E. III, editors. *Ethical Considerations in Long-Term Care*. Proceedings of a conference sponsored by the Geriatric Research, Education and Clinical Center, Veterans Administration Center, Bay Pines, Florida and Eckerd College of Gerontology Center, St. Petersburg, Fla., Suncoast Printing.

Wohleber, D. L. "Handling conflicts of interest." *Hospital Financial Management* 31(4):38-40, April 1977.

Wrenn, K. "No insurance, no admission." *New England Journal of Medicine* 312(6):373-374, February 7, 1985.

Yezzi, Ronald. *Medical Ethics: Thinking About Unavoidable Questions*. New York: Holt, Rinehart and Winston, 1980.

Youell, Linda. "Major ethical problems faced by nursing administrators." Major paper. Edmonton, Alberta: University of Alberta, 1984.

Youell, Linda. "A question of balance." *Canadian Nurse/ L'infirmiere canadienne* 82(3):26-30, 33, March 1986.

Youngner, S. J., D. L. Jackson, C. Coulten, B. W. Juknialis and E. M. Smith. "A national survey of hospital ethics committees." *Critical Care Medicine* 11(11):902-905, November 1983.

Zenisek, T. J. "Corporate social responsibility: a conceptualization based on organizational literature." *Academy of Management Review* 4(3):359-368, 1979.